Intention-Controlled Hand Rehabilitation for Stroke Survivors

Min Li · Bo He

Intention-Controlled Hand Rehabilitation for Stroke Survivors

Motion Assistance and Haptic Stimulation

西安交通大學出版社
XI'AN JIAOTONG UNIVERSITY PRESS

Springer

Min Li
School of Mechanical Engineering
Xi'an Jiaotong University
Xi'an, Shaanxi, China

Bo He
School of Mechanical Engineering
Xi'an Jiaotong University
Xi'an, Shaanxi, China

ISBN 978-981-95-4195-9 ISBN 978-981-95-4196-6 (eBook)
https://doi.org/10.1007/978-981-95-4196-6

Jointly published with Xi'an Jiaotong University Press.
The print edition is not for sale in China (Mainland). Customers from China (Mainland) please order the print book from: Xi'an Jiaotong University Press.

This Springer imprint is published by the registered company Springer Nature Singapore Pte Ltd.
The registered company address is: 152 Beach Road, #21-01/04 Gateway East, Singapore 189721, Singapore

Preface

Stroke remains one of the most pressing global health challenges, leaving millions with life-altering motor impairments—particularly in the hands, whose intricate functionality is pivotal to daily independence. Despite advances in rehabilitation, many survivors struggle to regain fine motor control, and traditional therapies often fall short in engaging patients actively or adapting to individual needs. This monograph emerges from a pressing need to bridge this gap: to translate cutting-edge research at the intersection of neuroscience, robotics, and human-computer interaction into practical, intent-driven solutions for hand rehabilitation.

Over the past decade, our team has explored how technology can amplify the brain's inherent capacity for neuroplasticity. We have sought to answer a critical question: *How can we design systems that not only assist movement but also align with a patient's intent, making rehabilitation an active, immersive process rather than a passive one?* This book synthesizes our findings, presenting a cohesive framework for intent-controlled hand rehabilitation that integrates wearable robotics, brain-computer interfaces (BCIs), and multisensory feedback—with a particular focus on the transformative role of fingertip haptic stimulation.

Readers will find a journey through five interconnected pillars of innovation:

- **Soft wearable exoskeletons** that mimic natural hand kinematics, prioritizing safety and adaptability for diverse users;
- **Bilateral training systems** that leverage the unimpaired hand's signals to guide the affected limb, addressing muscle synergy imbalances;
- **Tau-jerk motion planning** to optimize trajectories, minimizing compensatory movements and enhancing task relevance;
- **Attention-controlled BCIs** using low-cost EEG, making active engagement accessible beyond specialized labs;
- **Haptic feedback integration** that synchronizes tactile stimulation with movement, strengthening the sensorimotor loop critical for recovery.

Each chapter balances theory and practice, combining neurophysiological insights with experimental data, case studies, and technical designs. We delve into the challenges—from feedback latency to individual variability—and propose actionable solutions, supported by validation with human subjects.

This work is intended for a multidisciplinary audience: researchers in rehabilitation robotics and neuroscience will find novel methodologies for intent detection and feedback design; clinicians will gain insights into translating technology into patient-centric therapy; engineers will discover practical approaches to building affordable, user-friendly devices. Together, we hope it fosters collaboration across fields, accelerating the shift from passive assistance to active, intent-driven rehabilitation.

The road to restoring hand function after stroke is deeply personal, varying with each patient's neural resilience and life circumstances. Our goal is not to offer a one-size-fits-all solution, but to provide a toolkit of evidence-based strategies that honor this individuality. As technology continues to evolve, we believe the future of rehabilitation lies in systems that listen—to the brain's signals, the body's needs, and the patient's goals.

It is our hope that this book inspires further innovation, bringing us closer to a world where every stroke survivor can reclaim the ability to grasp, touch, and interact with life on their own terms.

Xi'an, China
2025

Min Li
Bo He

Acknowledgments

We express our deepest gratitude to our colleagues at the School of Mechanical Engineering, Xi'an Jiaotong University, for their invaluable support throughout this project. Special thanks to Prof. Guanghua Xu, Dr. Jun Xie, Prof. Tangfei Tao, and Prof. Sicong Zhang for their guidance and encouragement.

We are profoundly thankful to the dedicated students from our research group, including Jiazhou Chen, Guoying He, Jing Chen, Ziting Liang, Tianci Wang, Yueyan Zhuo, Shiqi Yang, Shengchen Zhu, Zhilei Shi, Yanjun Jia, Chaozhou Zhang, and Shufang Zheng. Their prior contributions at XJTU have laid a solid foundation for this book, and their unwavering support and collaboration have been integral to its completion.

We are grateful to Prof. Kaspar Althoefer from Queen Mary University of London for his exceptional mentorship to Dr. Min Li and for his continued collaboration even after her graduation.

We extend our appreciation to our collaborators Prof. Hua Yuan and Dr. Chen-Guang Zhao for providing essential medical insights that enriched the studies presented in this book.

Our heartfelt thanks also go to our collaborators and friends for their contributions and support: Prof. Chaoyang Chen from Wayne State University, Dr. Jichun Li from Newcastle University, Dr. Lei Cui from Curtin University, Emanuele Lindo Secco from Liverpool Hope University, Prof. Helge Wurdemann from University College London, Dr. Wei Yao from the University of Salford, and Dr. Sina Sareh and Prof. Paul Anderson from the Royal College of Art.

This work was made possible with partial funding from several organizations, including:

- The National Natural Science Foundation of China (Grants 51505363, 51775417, 51975451, and 52575344).
- The RSE–NSFC Joint Project (Grant 51911530243).
- The China Postdoctoral Science Foundation (Grants 2015M570821 and 2019M653586).

- The Natural Science Foundation of Shaanxi Province of China (Grants 2019JQ-332 and 2023-YBGY-353).
- The Key Research and Development Program of Shaanxi (Grant 2023-YBGY-353).
- The Guangdong S&T Programme (Grant 2015B020214001).
- The Fundamental Research Funds for the Central Universities (Grant xzy012019012).

Finally, we extend our sincere gratitude to all participants of the experiments, whose involvement was crucial for the success of our research.

Contents

Abbreviations

ADLs	Activities of Daily Living
ANOVA	Analysis of Variance
BCI	Brain-Computer Interface
BMI	Brain-Machine Interface
BP	Bereitschaftspotential
CMC	Carpometacarpal (Joint)
CPM	Continuous Passive Motion
DIP	Distal Interphalangeal (Joint)
DOF	Degree of Freedom
EEG	Electroencephalography
EMG	Electromyography
EOG	Electrooculography
ERP	Event-Related Potential
FES	Functional Electrical Stimulation
FMA	Fugl-Meyer Assessment
fMRI	Functional Magnetic Resonance Imaging
fNIRS	Functional Near-Infrared Spectroscopy
HG-C1100	Panasonic Laser Displacement Sensor Model
ICA	Independent Component Analysis
IP	Interphalangeal (Joint)
IPMC	Ionic Polymer Metal Composite
M1	Primary Motor Cortex
MAV	Mean Absolute Value
MCP	Metacarpophalangeal (Joint)
MEG	Magnetoencephalography
MEPs	Motor-Evoked Potentials
MI	Motor Imagery
MRCPs	Movement-Related Cortical Potentials
MRI	Magnetic Resonance Imaging
MVC	Maximum Voluntary Contraction
NMES	Neuromuscular Electrical Stimulation

OML	Vicon Motion Systems (Company)
P300	Event-Related Potential Component (300ms latency)
PD	Proportional-Derivative (Controller)
PI	Proportional-Integral (Controller)
PID	Proportional-Integral-Derivative (Controller)
PIP	Proximal Interphalangeal (Joint)
PPG	Photoplethysmography
RMS	Root Mean Square
ROM	Range of Motion
S1	Primary Somatosensory Cortex
SEM	Standard Error of the Mean
SMC	SMC Corporation (Pneumatic Components)
SPECT	Single-Photon Emission Computed Tomography
SSC	Slope Sign Change
SSMVEP	Steady-State Motion Visual Evoked Potential
SSVEP	Steady-State Visual Evoked Potential
SWMT	Semmes-Weinstein Monofilament Test
tACS	Transcranial Alternating Current Stimulation
tDCS	Transcranial Direct Current Stimulation
TMS	Transcranial Magnetic Stimulation
TST	Triple Stimulation Technique
WL	Waveform Length
ZC	Zero Crossing

Chapter 1
Motor Rehabilitation After Stroke: Neurophysiological Mechanisms and Human Intent-Controlled Approaches

Strokes remain a leading cause of acquired disability worldwide, demanding innovative interventions to restore motor function in survivors. This chapter synthesizes advances in human intent-controlled rehabilitation, a paradigm that bridges motor intent detection, peripheral stimulation, and neuroplasticity-driven recovery for stroke-affected hands. Beginning with the neurophysiological basis of intent-driven rehabilitation, we critically analyze state-of-the-art technologies for detecting movement intent—including electromyography (EMG), kinematics, and brain–machine interfaces (BMIs)—and their integration with assistive robotics and haptic feedback systems. We further explore quantitative motor assessment frameworks and address persistent challenges such as patient-specific variability, feedback latency, and clinical scalability. By emphasizing the interplay between intent detection, motion assistance, and sensory stimulation, this chapter sets the foundation for subsequent studies that advance hand rehabilitation through soft robotics, bilateral training, and multimodal haptic interfaces.

1.1 Introduction

Strokes are a major contributor to acquired disabilities globally, presenting significant challenges for individuals and healthcare systems alike (World Health Organization 2020). These cerebrovascular events occur due to the rupture or blockage of blood vessels in the brain, leading to cell death and disruptions in neural circuits (Ang and Guan 2013). The extent and location of brain lesions caused by stroke directly influence the severity of motor and sensory impairments (Ang and Guan 2013). Individuals who survive a stroke frequently encounter significant physical and cognitive obstacles, as impaired communication between the brain and body hampers their capacity to carry out essential daily tasks. Alarmingly, only a small percentage of survivors can resume professional activities, and over 30% require assistance for

M. Li and B. He, *Intention-Controlled Hand Rehabilitation for Stroke Survivors*,
https://doi.org/10.1007/978-981-95-4196-6_1

activities of daily living (ADLs) due to persistent functional impairments (Wurzinger et al. 2021).

Stroke rehabilitation focuses on regaining autonomy and enhancing overall well-being. This requires an interdisciplinary approach that combines neuroscience, robotics, computer science, and clinical methodologies (Wade and Winstein 2012). A critical factor in successful motor recovery is neuroplasticity—the brain's ability to adapt and reorganize itself (Li et al. 2018). Activating neuroplasticity through motor intent training has emerged as a promising avenue for rehabilitation (Norman et al. 2022). Human intent-controlled rehabilitation refers to therapeutic interventions that actively leverage a patient's residual motor intention—the conscious or subconscious neural drive to initiate or execute movement—to guide assistive devices or sensory feedback systems. Unlike passive therapies, where external devices or therapists mobilize limbs without requiring patient engagement (e.g., continuous passive motion machines), intent-controlled systems demand active participation. These systems detect movement intent through modalities such as EMG, electroencephalography (EEG), or kinematic sensors, then translate it into real-time assistance via robotic exoskeletons, functional electrical stimulation (FES), or haptic interfaces. By aligning therapeutic actions with the patient's internal motor commands, this approach reinforces efferent (brain-to-muscle) and afferent (sensory feedback-to-brain) pathways, thereby harnessing neuroplasticity to rebuild disrupted motor circuits. In contrast to passive methods, which prioritize repetitive motion alone, intent-controlled rehabilitation emphasizes *volitional engagement*, fostering cortical reorganization and functional recovery by ensuring that movements are purposeful, patient-driven, and contextually relevant to activities of daily living (ADLs). This paradigm shift not only enhances motor relearning but also empowers patients by restoring agency over their rehabilitation process.

Techniques like brain–machine interfaces (BMIs) facilitate this process by linking motor intent with sensory feedback, bypassing impaired movement pathways and stimulating the motor cortex (Donati et al. 2016). Studies suggest that active motor intent, paired with sensorimotor feedback, can drive more substantial neuroplastic changes compared to passive approaches (Mrachacz-Kersting et al. 2012; Takeuchi and Izumi 2013).

This chapter focuses on hand rehabilitation, where intent-controlled systems face unique challenges due to the hand's biomechanical complexity and the precision required for ADLs. The following points are reviewed:

- The neurophysiological basis of intent-driven motor recovery,
- Technologies for detecting and interpreting hand movement intent,
- Strategies for integrating intent with peripheral stimulation (e.g., haptic feedback, robotic assistance),
- Quantitative frameworks for assessing recovery in hand function.

The critical barriers to clinical adoption are also identified, including cognitive-motor decoupling in patients, system latency, and the need for personalized adaptive control. At the end of this chapter, it introduces the studies detailed in subsequent chapters that attempt to partially address the identified challenges.

1.2 Neurophysiological Foundations of Intent-Controlled Hand Rehabilitation

Neuroplasticity and Active Training in Hand Recovery

Neuroplasticity—the dynamic capability of the brain to remodel itself following exposure to new experiences—is central to restoring hand function after stroke. For the hand, which occupies a disproportionately large somatotopic area in the motor cortex (M1) and somatosensory cortex (S1), this adaptability is critical for relearning fine motor skills like grasping, pinching, and object manipulation (Johansson 2011; Pascual-Leone et al. 2011). Cortical remapping in post-stroke recovery occurs through three phases (Takeuchi and Izumi 2013; Langhorne et al. 2011):

- **Restitution**: Partial regeneration of neural networks in peri-infarct regions, particularly in the hand knob area of M1, which governs finger movements (Wieloch and Nikolich 2006).
- **Substitution**: Recruitment of adjacent cortical areas (e.g., premotor cortex) or contralateral hemispheres to compensate for lost hand function (Warraich and Kleim 2010).
- **Compensation**: Behavioral adaptation using alternative strategies (e.g., over-reliance on wrist flexion for grasping) (Langhorne et al. 2011; Warraich and Kleim 2010).

However, neuroplasticity can lead to maladaptive reorganization in the hand, such as abnormal flexor synergies (e.g., "clenched fist" postures) or sensory neglect, which hinder functional recovery (Dietz and Fouad 2014; Moxon et al. 2014). To counteract this, intent-controlled rehabilitation leverages activity-dependent plasticity by aligning assistive devices (e.g., soft robotic gloves, haptic interfaces) with the patient's residual motor intent. For example, EMG-driven exoskeletons amplify weakened finger movements while providing proprioceptive feedback, reinforcing efferent (motor command) and afferent (sensory) pathways (Piggott et al. 2016; Saposnik and Ovbiagele 2016). This closed-loop engagement mimics natural hand use, activating reward systems (e.g., dopaminergic pathways) that strengthen motor learning (Ethier et al. 2015; Ramos-Murguialday et al. 2013).

Mirror neuron systems further enhance hand-specific neuroplasticity. Observing or imagining hand movements—such as grasping a cup—activates M1 and premotor regions, priming the brain for relearning (Oztop et al. 2013). When combined with intent-controlled technologies like brain–computer interfaces (BCIs) or virtual reality (VR), these strategies improve hand function by simulating task-specific contexts (e.g., reaching in VR environments) (Park and Hwangbo 2015; Pichiorri et al. 2015). Critically, synchronized feedback (e.g., haptic cues timed to finger extension) is essential: delays exceeding 100 ms disrupt sensorimotor integration, reducing therapeutic efficacy (Grosse-Wentrup et al. 2011).

Thus, effective hand rehabilitation requires:

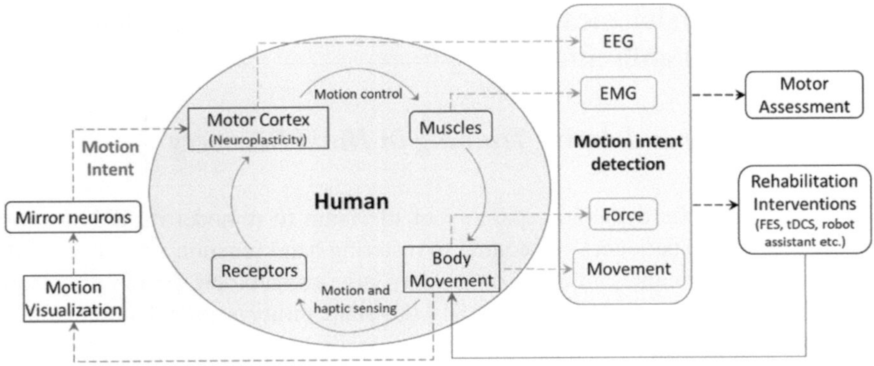

Fig. 1.1 Diagram of a motor rehabilitation system for stroke survivors controlled by human intent

- **Volitional Engagement**: Active initiation of movements (e.g., finger flexion detected via EMG/kinematics).
- **Task-Specific Practice**: ADL-oriented tasks (e.g., buttoning, utensil use) to drive cortical reorganization.
- **Multisensory Feedback**: Haptic, visual, and proprioceptive cues to reinforce correct motor patterns.

An illustrative diagram of this method is depicted in Fig. 1.1.

Sensory Integration in Hand Motor Recovery

The hand's dense concentration of mechanoreceptors (e.g., Merkel cells, Pacinian corpuscles) and proprioceptive fibers makes it uniquely dependent on sensory feedback for dexterity. Post-stroke sensory deficits—such as loss of two-point discrimination or grip-force modulation—disrupt the sensorimotor loop, leading to compensatory, inefficient movements (e.g., excessive grip force during object manipulation) (Umeda et al. 2019; Yu et al. 2022).

Sensorimotor integration (SMI) in hand recovery involves:

- **Afferent Pathways**: Sensory signals from fingertips (e.g., texture, pressure) ascend via the spinothalamic and dorsal column-medial lemniscus pathways to S1.
- **Cortical Processing**: S1 integrates tactile input with M1 motor commands, enabling precise grip control.
- **Efferent Adjustment**: M1 refines movements based on sensory feedback (e.g., adjusting finger position to prevent object slippage) (Umeda et al. 2019).

Stroke-induced damage to thalamocortical circuits disrupts this loop, causing sensory-motor decoupling. For example, impaired proprioception leads to "sensory ataxia," where patients overshoot or undershoot hand movements despite intact motor pathways (Macdonell et al. 1989). Rehabilitation must therefore address both motor and sensory deficits. Techniques like haptic stimulation (e.g., vibrotactile feedback during grasping) or sensorized gloves restore sensory input, while mirror therapy leverages visual feedback to "trick" the brain into perceiving movement in the affected hand (Park and Hwangbo 2015; Joshua 2022).

Multimodal sensory reinforcement is particularly powerful for the hand:

- **Tactile-Kinematic Synergy**: Combining fingertip vibration with robotic-assisted finger flexion improves grip-force modulation (Park and Hwangbo 2015; Ricciardi et al. 2007).
- **Cross-Modal Plasticity**: Auditory cues (e.g., clicking sounds during pinch tasks) enhance S1–M1 connectivity in chronic stroke patients (Solo-Faraco et al. 2004).

1.3 Techniques for Detecting Human Movement Intent in Hand Rehabilitation

Detecting human movement intent is a cornerstone of effective rehabilitation and can be achieved through various methods, including measuring interactive movements and forces between humans and machines (Patel et al. 2015; Castellini and Koiva 2013), analyzing EMG signals, or leveraging BCI technologies. This section focuses on EMG- and BCI-based techniques that enable precise, adaptive control of assistive devices (e.g., robotic gloves, exoskeletons) while integrating haptic feedback to reinforce sensorimotor pathways.

EMG-Based Detection for Hand Motor Control

EMG signals, which reflect neuromuscular activation, are widely used to detect intent for finger and wrist movements. In hand rehabilitation, surface EMG sensors are strategically placed on forearm flexor/extensor muscles to decode grasp/release intent (e.g., palmar versus lateral grip) (Batzianoulis et al. 2018). A feedback latency of under 200 ms is generally considered optimal in hand rehabilitation, ensuring the timeliness required for neuro-plasticity (Höhler et al. 2023). Compared to BCI methods, EMG signals can capture finer motor movements.

However, the reliability of EMG signals in stroke patients is often compromised due to muscle weakness, paralysis, and pathological synergies (Wright et al. 2014). Prolonged reliance on EMG for control might inadvertently reinforce pathological movements instead of fostering normal motor patterns (Krebs et al. 2003). To improve sensitivity and reliability of the EMG-based intention detection, adaptive algorithms (Özgünen et al. 2010; Ding et al. 2021) and high-density EMG arrays (Rojas-Martínez et al. 2020) have been explored.

BCI-Based Detection for Cortical Engagement

BCIs also known as BMIs, bypass impaired peripheral pathways, directly linking cortical activity to assistive devices—ideal for patients with severe hand paralysis, facilitating motor function relearning, promoting brain reorganization to compensate for lost functionality, and serving as neuromodulatory systems (Ang and Guan 2013; Wolpaw et al. 2002; Jiang et al. 2014a, b).

To acquire neural signals, BCIs can utilize various neuroimaging modalities, categorized into invasive and non-invasive approaches. Invasive methods encompass electrocorticography (ECoG) using subdural electrodes and direct intracortical neuron recording (Vansteensel et al. 2016). Less intrusive alternatives, which are more commonly used in rehabilitation contexts, include EEG, functional magnetic resonance imaging (fMRI), magnetoencephalography (MEG), single-photon emission computed tomography (SPECT), functional near-infrared spectroscopy (fNIRS), and positron emission tomography (PET) (Crosson et al. 2010).

When selecting a modality, factors such as usability, cost, and resolution of neural activity play critical roles (Dokkum et al. 2015). MEG and fMRI provide high-resolution data but are limited by their bulky equipment and operational constraints. In contrast, fNIRS offers a more practical alternative, with advantages such as portability, resistance to head motion artifacts, and the ability to perform in naturalistic settings without requiring MRI-compatible devices (Su et al. 2023). Recent studies have explored the use of fNIRS-based BCIs in rehabilitation settings. For instance, a 2023 study introduced an fNIRS-based MI training aiming at hand rehabilitation (Lyukmanov et al. 2024). These studies indicate ongoing advancements in fNIRS-based BCIs for rehabilitation, though the field is still developing.

EEG stands out as the most widely used signal for BCI research due to its non-invasiveness, portability, and ease of use (Nicolas-Alonso and Gomez-Gil 2012). The modalities of EEG that can be used for hand specific intent detection are shown in the following paragraphs.

Motor Imagery (MI) MI induces event-related desynchronization (ERD) and synchronization (ERS) in the sensorimotor oscillations, reflecting neural activation patterns associated with movement preparation and execution (Vuckovic and Osuagwu 2013). MI allows for the real-time categorization of neuroelectric brain activity, enabling the prediction of when a movement will occur, its direction, and even which limb will be involved. Recent advancements in MI research have demonstrated its ability to predict movement parameters such as trajectory, force, and timing, expanding its applications in neurorehabilitation and BCIs (Benzy et al. 2020; Gatti et al. 2021). However, one limitation of MI-based BCIs is that users typically require prior training before their neural signals can be reliably interpreted. Moreover, the accuracy of intention decoding depends strongly on the user's concentration and their ability to consistently and accurately perform motor imagery tasks (Li et al. 2015). Novel training approaches, such as adaptive neurofeedback systems and gamified environments, have shown promise in enhancing user engagement and reducing training time (Hadjiaros et al. 2023). For stroke survivors, alterations in ERD/ERS responses may limit the effectiveness of MI-based rehabilitation (Teo and Chew 2014). Object-oriented MI, which incorporates task-specific imagery, have been shown to better activate the mirror neuron system, fostering improved motor imagery ability and neural plasticity (Liang et al. 2016). Furthermore, integrating multimodal sensory stimuli—such as auditory, visual, and haptic cues—has demonstrated synergistic effects on activating mirror neurons and enhancing MI performance (Zschorlich et al. 2021; Su et al. 2024). Neuromodulation techniques such as transcranial alternating current stimulation (tACS) and transcranial direct current stimulation (tDCS) have been found to potentiate ERD responses, resulting in improved MI accuracy (Ang et al. 2012; Kasashima et al. 2012). Additionally, the emergence of closed-loop neuromodulation systems offers new possibilities for tailoring stimulation to individual neural states in real time (Wahl et al. 2023). Finally, recent advances in high-resolution EEG and machine learning-based analysis have enhanced the precision of temporal motor intent detection, enabling more reliable integration of MI-based systems into practical applications (Sharma et al. 2023; Zhang et al. 2022).

Studies using ERD/ERS-based neuromodulation has seldom documented the precise timing of motor intent detection.

Movement-Related Cortical Potentials (MRCPs) MRCPs are considered direct and dependable markers of cortical changes occurring during motor skill acquisition (Yilmaz et al. 2015). The Bereitschaftspotential (BP), a significant component of MRCPs, typically begins 1–2 s before motion onset, offering a predictive window for movement intent (Ahmadian et al. 2013). This characteristic has been leveraged in rehabilitation strategies, such as MRCP-based BCI triggering robot-assisted motor training in seven post-stroke patients with hand impairment (Butt et al. 2021). Although naive subjects can produce MRCP signals in their first session without prior training, the need for calibration (training) in MRCP-based BCIs is still viewed as a limitation due to the variability between trials (Bhagat et al. 2016). To promote the practical application of BCIs in clinical environments, it is important to reduce the time needed for system setup, sensor calibration, and user training. Therefore, research has focused on enhancing the performance of MRCP-based BCIs by improving detection accuracy, reducing latency, addressing trial-to-trial variability, and reducing cost (Said et al. 2022; Gulyás and Jochumsen 2024).

MRCPs allow for the detection of movement-related neural activity with a latency ranging from approximately − 600 to 500 ms relative to movement onset (Bhagat et al. 2016; Niazi et al. 2012; Xu et al. 2014).

Motion Visual Evoked Potentials (mVEPs) Human motor intention can also be triggered by visual stimuli. mVEPs are measurable in the visual cortex after the display of visual stimuli and hold significant potential for investigating how individuals perceive and interpret motion-related information (Hong et al. 2009). Various SSMVEP-based stimulation paradigms have been developed for BCI applications (Yan et al. 2017; Xie et al. 2012). They typically involve a visual movement stimulus first, followed by the individual's perception of the motion. BCIs that utilize SSMVEP determine the focused stimulus being attended to by comparing the frequency components in the neural signals with the movement frequency of the visual cue. Consequently, the individual's motion intent can be detected. This type of BCI achieves a detection accuracy exceeding 88% (Karimi et al. 2022; Zhang et al. 2021), supported by improvements in stimulus design and signal processing. Hybrid visual stimuli that combine periodic motion elements with traditional flickering or pattern-reversal visual stimuli have been proposed to evoke stronger and more distinguishable VEP responses, leading to improved classification accuracy (Kwon et al. 2022).

The time components consist of stimulation duration (around 300 ms), visual processing latency (~140 ms), and online computation time (roughly 80 ms) (Chen et al. 2015).

Hybrid Systems for Robust Hand Control

Hybrid systems integrate complementary signals to address the limitations of single-modality approaches, enhancing control accuracy, adaptability, and robustness.

- **Hybrid BCI**: Hybrid-BCI systems integrate at least two distinct neurophysiological signals or acquisition modalities to enhance performance and versatility. For instance, combining ERD and SSMVEP leverages complementary neural mechanisms for improved intent detection (Zhang et al. 2021). These systems also merge diverse signal types, such as functional near-infrared spectroscopy (fNIRS) and EEG, to exploit the synergistic strengths of them. A notable example is the work by Ortega and Faisal (Ortega and Faisal 2021), who developed a hybrid BCI using EEG and fNIRS to decode bimanual grip force. Their approach employed a deep-learning architecture with attention mechanisms and residual layers, optimizing multimodal signal fusion and achieving superior decoding accuracy. Compared to single-modality BCIs, hybrid systems offer expanded control capabilities, higher information transfer rates, and enhanced robustness against noise—critical advantages for real-world applications in complex tasks like hand rehabilitation (Pfurtscheller 2010).
- **EMG–EEG Fusion**: The integration of EMG and EEG creates a synergistic framework that expands the scope of control commands beyond the limitations of individual modalities (Zhang et al. 2019). EMG provides high-resolution detection of muscle activity, enabling precise tracking of peripheral motor execution, while EEG captures cortical intent, reflecting the brain's preparatory and planning signals (Yang et al. 2023; Cho et al. 2022). This hybrid approach is particularly advantageous for decoding complex tasks, such as individuated finger movements or force modulation during grasping. For example, Chowdhury et al. (2019) developed a corticomuscular feature extraction approach that relies on the relationship between power fluctuations within specific frequency bands over time from EMG and EEG signals to identify task-specific neural-muscular coupling. By analyzing synchronized cortical and muscular activity, their algorithm achieved

robust single-trial classification of motor tasks. Such advancements underscore the potential of EMG–EEG fusion to refine adaptive control of assistive devices (e.g., robotic gloves) in stroke rehabilitation, where precise alignment of cortical intent and muscle activation is critical for restoring functional hand movements.

- **Multimodal Sensor Fusion**: These systems enhance intent detection by integrating complementary modalities, such as EMG with force sensors for grip pressure measurement or inertial measurement units (IMUs) for motion tracking (Wright et al. 2014; Ghassemi et al. 2019). Similarly, EEG can be combined with non-neural modalities like motion capture (Cho et al. 2022) and eye tracking (Chowdhury et al. 2019) to provide richer contextual information. By resolving ambiguities in neural signals—such as differentiating between idle states and movement preparation—and incorporating task-specific context, multimodal fusion significantly improves control accuracy. For example, motion capture validates EEG-predicted hand trajectories, while eye tracking anticipates grasp patterns by identifying visual targets. These integrations are particularly valuable in hand rehabilitation, where precise, spatiotemporal coordination of finger movements is critical for effective motor recovery.

Advancements in machine learning now enable seamless multimodal signal integration, allowing adaptive responses to diverse user needs and environmental conditions. These intelligent fusion techniques have demonstrated superior performance in motor control tasks, paving the way for practical applications in neurorehabilitation and assistive technology. For example, Luo et al. (2023) developed a hybrid BCI that integrates MI with steady-state visual evoked potentials (SSVEP) in a unified system using a convolutional neural network (CNN). This system autonomously extracts EEG features from both paradigms, improving decoding accuracy by 2.6% compared to SSVEP alone and 25.4% compared to MI alone. The effectiveness of this approach was validated across both single and hybrid-mode scenarios, underscoring its potential for real-world neurorehabilitation applications.

1.4 Intent-Controlled Peripheral Stimulation

This section explores how aligning human intent with peripheral stimulation enhances hand motor recovery in stroke survivors. We focus on modalities that leverage intent detection (e.g., EMG, EEG) to deliver targeted, adaptive feedback, emphasizing applications for hand-specific rehabilitation.

Electrical, Magnetic, and Sensory Stimulation Methods

Electrical Stimulation and Magnetic Stimulation

Neuromuscular electrical stimulation (NMES) is a well-established approach for stroke rehabilitation, triggering the depolarization of peripheral nerve cells to induce muscle contractions. This promotes neuroplastic modifications and improves motor function (Quandt and Hummel 2014). Functional electrical stimulation (FES), a related technique, stimulates nerves or motor points in a structured order to generate movements resembling voluntary motions (Borroni and Baldissera 2008). Intent-controlled FES, leveraging signals from EMG (Lu et al. 2023; Ambrosini et al. 2021) or EEG (Zulauf-Czaja et al. 2021), has shown significant promise in active rehabilitation training by enhancing neuroplasticity and improving motor recovery (Nojima et al. 2022; Bai et al. 2020).

Transcranial direct current stimulation (tDCS) employs mild polarizing currents to influence cortical activity, adjusting brain excitability either upwards or downwards (Nitsche and Paulus 2000). When combined with MI-BCIs and robotic feedback, tDCS has demonstrated improved rehabilitation outcomes, particularly in enhancing MI effectiveness for upper-limb recovery (Ang and Guan 2013). However, contrasting findings, such as those by Hu et al. (2021), suggest that tDCS and MI-BCI might have varying or even contradictory impacts on post-stroke cortical reorganization, indicating the need for further investigation into optimal protocols.

Transcranial magnetic stimulation (TMS) utilizes magnetic fields to adjust cortical responsiveness, aiming to restore interhemispheric balance by increasing excitability in the affected motor cortex and reducing activity in the intact side. MI (ERD)-controlled TMS has been proven to increase corticospinal responsiveness and support motor recovery, as demonstrated by Kraus et al. (2016). Further applications include using MI-controlled TMS to explore corticocortical contributions to motor imagery tasks (Levy et al. 2016). However, the need to recalibrate cranial targets for each session remains a limitation of TMS-based therapies.

Epidural electrical stimulation (EECS), when combined with task-oriented upper-limb rehabilitation, has shown superior outcomes compared to rehabilitation alone (Levy et al. 2016). EECS targets cortical and spinal pathways, reinforcing plasticity and enhancing the effects of traditional therapies.

Sensory Feedback for Motor Rehabilitation

Visual Stimulation Visual feedback plays a key role in stroke rehabilitation by enhancing patients' confidence and facilitating motor learning. Visualizing outputs such as force or EMG activity activates the mirror neuron system and recruits action observation networks, engaging motor and premotor cortices. Abstract and naturalistic visualizations have both been effective in stimulating cortical activity. However, visual feedback may not be suitable for patients with impaired vision.

Auditory Stimulation For visually impaired patients, auditory stimulation provides an alternative feedback modality. Compared to visual stimulation, auditory cues lessen the perceptual and cognitive burden while minimizing distractions, making them particularly effective in rehabilitation tasks (Helmer et al. 2011; Secoli et al. 2011). However, when conveying complex information using auditory cues, cognitive load will also be increased (Bastola et al. 2023).

Haptic Feedback Haptic feedback utilizes the bidirectional nature of the somatosensory system to facilitate interaction with simulated environments, inducing neuroplasticity and reinforcing motor learning. Techniques such as position control, haptic guidance, and haptic-augmented environments strengthen muscles, reinforce movement patterns, and increase motivation (Marchal-Crespo and Reinkensmeyer 2009). Devices like the WAM robot arm (Barrett Technology, Inc.) provide advanced somatosensory feedback (Demain et al. 2013), although visual force feedback can substitute in the absence of dedicated haptic devices (Patel et al. 2015). Haptic guidance and assistance, typically robot-generated (Sigrist et al. 2013), will be explored in detail in Sect. 1.4.3.

Tactile Stimulation Tactile feedback, including vibrotactile feedback and percutaneous nerve stimulation, has shown potential in motor and tactile rehabilitation. For instance, Ganzer et al. (2020) developed a brain-controlled vibrotactile feedback system for spinal cord injury patients, while Geng et al. (2022) applied multi-point percutaneous nerve stimulation for peripheral nerve injury rehabilitation. These approaches demonstrate preliminary evidence of somatosensory cortical activation and improved tactile functions, although further research is needed to fully understand their efficacy in stroke rehabilitation.

Multisensory Integration

Stroke often results in sensory deficits, necessitating the integration of multiple feedback modalities to enhance recovery. The human brain processes sensory information from various modalities concurrently, with multisensory influences playing a crucial role in cortical functions (Johansson 2011). Multimodal feedback—combining visual, auditory, and haptic cues—has been shown to promote motor recovery effectively (Li et al. 2022a; Proulx et al. 2022). Combining BCI-FES with multimodal sensory feedback, including visual, somatosensory, and electro-tactile stimulation has been proposed to enhance task-specific outcomes (Remsik et al. 2022). VR and robotics provide versatile platforms for delivering integrated sensory feedback, creating immersive and engaging rehabilitation experiences.

Virtual Reality-Mediated Hand Rehabilitation

VR offers an immersive, multi-sensory environment that closely mimics real-world scenarios, providing users with instantaneous feedback on their actions. This feedback ensures movement accuracy without constant supervision from a therapist (Norris et al. 2024). Additionally, VR systems allow for the fine-tuning of settings, enabling personalized treatment plans tailored to individual needs. The versatility of VR facilitates its seamless integration with other therapeutic interventions, empowering researchers and clinicians to design patient-centric rehabilitation strategies that improve functional outcomes and the well-being of people living with neurological conditions (Ceradini et al. 2024).

Mechanisms of VR in Rehabilitation While most VR systems primarily deliver visual stimulation, many also incorporate auditory and tactile feedback to enhance user experience (Shi and Shen 2024). VR-based motor rehabilitation leverages several mechanisms, including neuroplasticity, engagement of the mirror neuron system, and activation of the neural circuitry associated with reward processing, all of which contribute to its efficacy in stroke recovery (Feitosa et al. 2022; Aderinto et al. 2023). The ability of VR to activate the mirror neuron system through motor observation is particularly significant. By visually perceiving movement, patients can stimulate the motor cortex, which maps this information to the primary somatosensory area, aiding in movement planning and execution (Park and Hwangbo 2015). Visual feedback also helps refine proprioceptive signals sent to the cerebral cortex, updating the body schema stored there and assisting in completing the "perception-processing-response" loop (Thøgersen et al. 2018).

Applications of VR in Motor Rehabilitation VR systems are uniquely capable of interpreting patient intent and adapting in real-time to create an interactive rehabilitation process. Recent advancements have explored the integration of BCIs with VR to facilitate motor rehabilitation. For instance, Gao et al. (2023) developed a hand rehabilitation platform integrating BCI technology, a soft robotic glove, and VR to aid stroke patients with hand movement disorders. In a study involving eleven stroke patients, experimental results showed that this BCI-driven rehabilitation system not only engaged a larger area of the cerebral cortex in the rehabilitation process but also improved muscle strength, reduced muscle tension, and enhanced overall hand motor function.

Challenges and Future Directions Despite its potential, VR-mediated rehabilitation faces challenges that need to be addressed for widespread clinical adoption. These include high costs, complex equipment requirements, patient suitability (e.g., sensory or cognitive impairments), data privacy concerns, and acceptance among patients and clinicians (Aderinto et al. 2023).

Robot-Based Hand Rehabilitation

Robot-based hand rehabilitation, also known as robot-assisted hand rehabilitation, utilizes advanced robotic systems that integrate sensory feedback, actuation mechanisms, and computational intelligence to support the recovery of motor functions (Ranzani et al. 2020). Such systems provide detailed kinetic and kinematic data during therapy sessions, enabling real-time performance analysis and adaptive responses based on metrics such as force, torque, joint angles, and positions. By tailoring interventions to individual patient needs, robot-assisted rehabilitation ensures a personalized and effective approach (Li et al. 2024; Gu et al. 2022). Machine learning algorithms (MLAs) further enhance this personalization by analyzing data trends and predicting future conditions, optimizing the rehabilitation process (Gu et al. 2022; Ai et al. 2023).

Repetitive Training and Neuroplasticity Central to robot-assisted rehabilitation is repetitive movement training, which emphasizes kinesthetic information, including speed, posture, and positional awareness, acquired through proprioception. This training stimulates the sensory-motor neurons in the cerebral cortex, enhancing the functional use of affected limbs and promoting brain plasticity. Over time, this approach supports sustained motor recovery and improves the overall rehabilitation outcomes (Hogan et al. 2006).

EMG-Driven Robot-Assisted Rehabilitation Robot-assisted systems have shown significant promise in clinical applications. Both trigger-type (Song et al. 2013a) and proportional control mechanisms (Song et al. 2013b) are widely used, offering flexible and intuitive control options. Additionally, motion pattern recognition based on EMG data has emerged as a sophisticated method for guiding robotic therapy, allowing for more precise and personalized interventions (Leonardis et al. 2015). For example, Chen et al. (2022) showed that therapy using EMG-driven robotic assistance was equally effective as task-focused training in improving hand and arm function during daily activities. Furthermore, this type of therapy demonstrated superior efficiency in enhancing movement duration for functional tasks.

BMI-Enabled Robot-Assisted Rehabilitation BMI-enabled robot-assisted rehabilitation combines robotic feedback with BCI technologies to facilitate motor recovery. Ang et al. (2010) demonstrated that integrating robotic feedback with EEG-based MI BCI significantly improved upper limb recovery in stroke survivors. Similarly, Varkuti et al. (2013) showed that MI EEG-BCI-based robotic therapy led to greater improvements in Fugl-Meyer assessment scores and enhanced functional brain connectivity compared to conventional robot-assisted methods. Recent research has expanded the capabilities of BMI-enabled systems by exploring other EEG features. These include SSVEP (Li et al. 2022b) and SSMVEP (Zhang et al. 2021). Such advancements aim to refine the precision and effectiveness of robot-assisted rehabilitation by leveraging richer neural data.

1.5 Assessing Motor Function in Intent-Controlled Hand Rehabilitation

Accurate assessment of motor function is pivotal for tailoring intent-driven rehabilitation strategies, particularly for the hand—a complex system requiring precision in grasp, force modulation, and dexterity. This section evaluates traditional and emerging methods, emphasizing hand-specific metrics and technologies aligned with modern rehabilitation paradigms.

Traditional Clinical Assessments Conventional assessment methods like the Fugl-Meyer Assessment (FMA) and the Action Research Arm Test (ARAT) rely heavily on therapist observations to evaluate tasks like pinch strength and finger individuation. While these scales serve as fundamental benchmarks in rehabilitation, they often lack the sensitivity needed to detect subtle improvements in fine motor skills, such as enhanced pincer grasp, and struggle to provide standardized outcomes across different therapeutic approaches (Resquín et al. 2016). The inherent subjectivity of therapist-dependent scoring introduces inter-rater variability, reducing consistency and reliability in patient evaluations (Zbytniewska et al. 2021). Furthermore, many traditional assessments focus on isolated movements rather than assessing how well patients integrate these motor improvements into functional daily activities (Zbytniewska et al. 2021). Their dependence on trained professionals also makes them time-consuming and less feasible for high-volume rehabilitation settings. Additionally, conventional tools primarily emphasize gross motor recovery while often neglecting critical aspects such as sensory re-education, proprioception, and neuromuscular adaptations. To address these gaps, sensory assessments like the Semmes–Weinstein Monofilament Test (SWMT) for tactile sensitivity, the Two-Point Discrimination Test for spatial acuity, and proprioceptive evaluations of joint position sense offer valuable complementary insights. Integrating these sensory assessments with conventional motor evaluations ensures a more comprehensive and precise understanding of sensorimotor recovery, ultimately leading to more effective rehabilitation strategies.

Automated and Wearable Sensor-Based Systems To address these limitations, automated assessment systems powered by machine learning algorithms (MLAs) have emerged (Ambros-Antemate et al. 2022). For example, Guo et al. (2022a) developed a system that analyzes hand movement data using a dynamic time warping algorithm to compare patients' movement patterns with standardized templates. Additionally, a mapping model based on the support vector regression (SVR) algorithm correlates movement data with clinical Fugl-Meyer Assessment (FMA) scores, providing objective evaluations of motor function. This approach reduces reliance on subjective therapist assessments and enhances consistency in patient evaluations. Beyond hand rehabilitation, machine learning has been widely applied to rehabilitation assessment across various domains. For instance, Jiang et al. (2023) developed a serious game that utilizes fuzzy logic to assess upper limb motor impairments by integrating motor performance data with therapist input. To ensure assessments reflect real-world functional reintegration, researchers are developing tasks that simulate daily activities and real-life scenarios (Altenburger et al. 2023). Such automated systems hold significant potential for complementing home-based rehabilitation, allowing patients to monitor their progress independently and engage in self-directed therapy more effectively.

Intent-adaptive rehabilitation programs necessitate precise, ongoing, and objective evaluation methods. Wearable sensors, modern motion capture technologies, and IoT connectivity facilitate continuous remote monitoring and objective assessment of human movement, providing invaluable insights into the neuromuscular abnormalities caused by strokes (Guo et al. 2022b; Porciuncula et al. 2018). Key variables such as joint synergy index (Ozturk et al. 2016), pinch strength (Patel et al. 2015), jerk metric and normalized jerk of standard movements (Turolla et al. 2013) are increasingly employed to offer a comprehensive understanding of motor function.

Neuromuscular Insights Via EMG EMG assessments further deepen understanding of neuromuscular impairments. Metrics like muscle activation levels (In et al. 2015), patterns of activation (Semprini et al. 2015), levels of co-contraction (Hu et al. 2015), complexity (Sun et al. 2014), and time-to-peak contractions (Fan et al. 2014) are pivotal in evaluating recovery. The concept of muscle synergies, which simplifies neuromuscular control, has recently gained traction as a promising approach for post-stroke assessment. For example, Scotto di Luzio et al. (2022) investigated the alteration of hand muscle synergies in stroke patients after robot-assisted rehabilitation. The researchers found that analyzing muscle synergies provided valuable insights into the neural control strategies of the hand post-stroke, highlighting its potential as an effective assessment tool in hand rehabilitation.

Neurophysiological Biomarkers Traditional behavioral metrics, while valuable, may fail to capture individual differences in brain structure and function during recovery (Leamy et al. 2014). Increasingly, physiological and neurological markers are being employed for more accurate motor function assessments. Technologies like EEG, fMRI, and NIRS offer direct insights into brain activity and cortical reorganization. Variability in EEG features among stroke patients with similar scores on conventional tests highlights the importance of individualized assessments (Tang et al. 2023). Advanced EEG metrics such as power spectral density analysis, oscillatory power suppression in the motor-associated cortex during MI (Jiang et al. 2015), and connectivity estimation (Pichiorri et al. 2015), have been used to evaluate brain function during rehabilitation. Additionally, techniques like Limpel-Zic complexity analysis (Gómez et al. 2016) provide nuanced assessments of brain states. Moreover, high-density EEG and ultra-high-field fMRI are enabling detailed mapping of brain activity, uncovering novel biomarkers for motor recovery (Sun et al. 2024). Other innovative approaches include NIRS-based cortical perfusion analysis (Zheng et al. 2023; Jiang et al. 2024) and fMRI measurements of cerebral blood volume changes before, during, and after rehabilitation (Ono et al. 2013).

Advanced Electrodiagnostics Electrodiagnostic techniques, such as nerve conduction studies and evoked potential analysis, are valuable tools for assessing the nervous system's integrity. Motor-evoked potentials (MEPs) elicited by TMS frequently employed to evaluate motor cortex excitability (Pichiorri et al. 2015; Kraus et al. 2016). The triple stimulation technique (TST) represents an enhanced approach to MEP assessment (Magistris et al. 1998). The TST, which combines TMS with peripheral electrical stimulation, offers an enhanced method to determine the proportion of activated spinal motor neurons, providing a detailed assessment of motor nerve conduction integrity. While TST is highly accurate, it faces challenges such as high costs, electromagnetic radiation exposure, and limited patient suitability (Rossi et al. 2009).

Multimodal Fusion and AI-Driven Analytics Integrating data from EEG, EMG, motion capture, and wearable sensors provides a holistic understanding of motor recovery (Xu et al. 2016). Multi-modal fusion algorithms combine cortical activity, muscle synergies, and biomechanical data for comprehensive assessment, providing a comprehensive understanding of motor function (Lorenz et al. 2024). Recent advancements in AI and deep learning models are enabling more accurate detection of subtle changes in motor function (Swarnakar and Yadav 2023).

1.6 Addressing Challenges and Future Directions

The clinical adoption of intent-controlled rehabilitation systems faces significant barriers, particularly for hand recovery. High costs and operational complexity, as seen in commercial BCI systems like those from g.tec, limit accessibility. To address this, researchers are prioritizing the development of affordable, non-invasive alternatives, such as dry EEG sensors and 3D-printed soft robotic gloves, which align with the need for scalable solutions. Personalization remains another critical challenge, as stroke survivors exhibit wide variability in EEG/EMG signals due to lesion location and severity. Adaptive algorithms that decode patient-specific neural and muscular patterns, such as attenuated sensorimotor rhythms or pathological muscle synergies, are essential for tailoring interventions (Leamy et al. 2014). Cognitive-motor decoupling further complicates BCI efficacy, as attention deficits in stroke patients reduce engagement with abstract feedback. Hybrid systems that integrate tactile or visual cues—like fingertip haptic stimulation or eye-tracking interfaces—may enhance participation by grounding intent in perceptible stimuli.

Integrative feedback mechanisms, such as pairing exoskeleton-assisted movements with synchronized vibrotactile cues, show promise in driving neuroplasticity. However, timing delays exceeding 300 ms between intent detection and robotic response can disrupt sensorimotor integration (Grosse-Wentrup et al. 2011; Wolters et al. 2003), underscoring the need for real-time closed-loop systems. Conflicting feedback priorities—such as competing visual, auditory, and haptic cues—also risk overwhelming patients. Emerging solutions dynamically adjust feedback weighting based on task demands; for example, prioritizing haptic signals during precision grips to refine force modulation. Deeper insights into cortical activation patterns across feedback modalities, particularly in hand-specific tasks, are needed to optimize these systems.

Multi-domain data fusion offers a pathway to precision rehabilitation. Studies leveraging transfer entropy reveal heightened EEG-EMG coherence in stroke patients during hand movements, reflecting compensatory neural recruitment. By integrating cortical intent (EEG), muscle activation (EMG), and kinematics, hybrid systems can decode grasp types while preventing maladaptive synergies. Machine learning models that synthesize these data streams identify latent recovery biomarkers, such as muscle synergy indices, enabling personalized therapy dosing.

1.7 Overview of Subsequent Chapters

In this chapter, it establishes the neurophysiological basis and core challenges of intent-controlled hand rehabilitation, laying groundwork for subsequent technologies. The following chapters expand on the neurophysiological principles and challenges outlined here, presenting innovative solutions tailored to hand rehabilitation.

From Chaps. 2 to 4, it talks about hardware innovations. Chapter 2 explores soft wearable robots, emphasizing 3D-printed gloves that assist finger abduction while prioritizing natural kinematics and affordability. Chapter 3 introduces bilateral rehabilitation systems that replicate the unimpaired hand's EMG signals to guide the affected limb, addressing muscle synergy imbalances. Chapter 4 optimizes exoskeleton finger trajectories using tau-jerk motion planning to minimize compensatory wrist movements, aligning with quantitative motor assessments. These three chapters covers the progresses from basic soft exoskeleton design (Chap. 2) to advanced control (bilateral systems, Chap. 3) and optimized motion planning (Chap. 4), focusing on aligning technology with natural human movement.

Chapters 5, 6, and 7 shift to enhancing patient participation via attention control and integrating fingertip haptic feedback, addressing cognitive-motor decoupling and sensory deficits. Chapter 5 leverages low-cost EEG sensors and gamified tasks to enhance attention-driven engagement, directly countering cognitive-motor decoupling. Chapters 6 and 7 synthesize motion assistance and haptic feedback into closed-loop systems, offering a unified framework for adaptive, multisensory rehabilitation. In Chap. 6, the role of fingertip haptic stimulation is investigated, showcasing its potential to improve attention activation during rehabilitation exercises. Chapter 7 investigates the combined benefits of integrating exoskeleton-supported hand rehabilitation with fingertip haptic feedback, aiming to enhance activation in both motor and sensory regions of the cortex during stroke rehabilitation through a comprehensive analysis involving both behavioral metrics and event-related potentials data.

Finally, Chap. 8 concludes by integrating insights from all chapters, identifying limitations, and outlining future directions.

Together, these chapters systematically address the technical, clinical, and mechanistic challenges of intent-controlled hand rehabilitation, advancing toward scalable, patient-centric solutions.

References

Aderinto N, Olatunji G, Abdulbasit MO et al (2023) Exploring the efficacy of virtual reality-based rehabilitation in stroke: a narrative review of current evidence. Ann Med 55:2285907. https://doi.org/10.1080/07853890.2023.2285907

Ahmadian P, Cagnoni S, Ascari L (2013) How capable is non-invasive EEG data of predicting the next movement ? A mini review. Front Hum Neurosci 7:1–7. https://doi.org/10.3389/fnhum.2013.00124

Ai Q, Liu Z, Meng W et al (2023) Machine learning in robot-assisted upper limb rehabilitation: a focused review. IEEE Trans Cogn Dev Syst 15:8350. https://doi.org/10.1109/TCDS.2021.3098350

Altenburger P, Ambike SS, Haddad JM (2023) Integrating motor variability evaluation into movement system assessment. Phys Ther 103:pzad075. https://doi.org/10.1093/ptj/pzad075

Ambros-Antemate JF, Reyes-Flores A, Argueta-Figueroa L et al (2022) Accuracy of machine learning algorithms for the assessment of upper-limb motor impairments in patients with post-stroke hemiparesis: a systematic review and meta-analysis. Adv Clin Exper Med 31:1309–1318

Ambrosini E, Gasperini G, Zajc J et al (2021) A robotic system with EMG-triggered functional electrical stimulation for restoring arm functions in stroke survivors. Neurorehabil Neural Repair 35:334–345. https://doi.org/10.1177/1545968321997769

Ang KK, Guan C, Chua KSG et al (2010) Clinical study of neurorehabilitation in stroke using EEG-based motor imagery brain–computer interface with robotic feedback. In: Proceedings of the 2010 annual international conference of the IEEE engineering in medicine and biology society, EMBC'10, pp 5549–5552

Ang KK, Guan C, Phua KS et al (2012) Transcranial direct current stimulation and EEG-based motor imagery BCI for upper limb stroke rehabilitation. In: Conference proceedings IEEE EMBS, pp 4128–4131

Ang KK, Guan C (2013) Brain–computer interface in stroke rehabilitation. J Comput Sci Eng 7:139–146. https://doi.org/10.5626/JCSE.2013.7.2.139

Bai Z, Fong KNK, Zhang JJ et al (2020) Immediate and long-term effects of BCI-based rehabilitation of the upper extremity after stroke: a systematic review and meta-analysis. J Neuroeng Rehabil 17:57. https://doi.org/10.1186/s12984-020-00686-2

Bastola A, Gluck A, Brinkley J (2023) Feedback mechanism for blind and visually impaired: a review. Proceed Hum Fact Ergon Soc Ann Meet 67:1748–1754. https://doi.org/10.1177/21695067231192448

Batzianoulis I, Krausz NE, Simon AM et al (2018) Decoding the grasping intention from electromyography during reaching motions. J Neuroeng Rehabil 15:57. https://doi.org/10.1186/s12984-018-0396-5

Benzy VK, Vinod AP, Subasree R et al (2020) Motor imagery hand movement direction decoding using brain computer interface to aid stroke recovery and rehabilitation. IEEE Trans Neural Syst Rehabil Eng 28:3051–3062. https://doi.org/10.1109/TNSRE.2020.3039331

Bhagat NA, Venkatakrishnan A, Abibullaev B et al (2016) Design and optimization of an EEG-based brain machine interface (BMI) to an upper-limb exoskeleton for stroke survivors. Front Neurosci 10:122. https://doi.org/10.3389/fnins.2016.00122

Borroni P, Baldissera F (2008) Activation of motor pathways during observation and execution of hand movements. Soc Neurosci 3:276–288. https://doi.org/10.1080/17470910701515269

Butt M, Naghdy G, Naghdy F et al (2021) Effect of robot-assisted training on EEG-derived movement-related cortical potentials for post-stroke rehabilitation: a case series study. IEEE Access 9:154143–154155. https://doi.org/10.1109/ACCESS.2021.3127939

Castellini C, Koiva R (2013) Using a high spatial resolution tactile sensor for intention detection. IEEE rehabilitation robotics (ICORR). IEEE, Seattle, pp 1–7

Ceradini M, Losanno E, Micera S et al (2024) Immersive VR for upper-extremity rehabilitation in patients with neurological disorders: a scoping review. J Neuroeng Rehabil 21:75. https://doi.org/10.1186/s12984-024-01367-0

Chen X, Wang Y, Nakanishi M et al (2015) High-speed spelling with a noninvasive brain–computer interface. Proceed Natl Acad Sci 112:E6058–E6067. https://doi.org/10.1073/pnas.1508080112

Chen Y-W, Chiang W-C, Chang C-L et al (2022) Comparative effects of EMG-driven robot-assisted therapy versus task-oriented training on motor and daily function in patients with stroke: a randomized cross-over trial. J Neuroeng Rehabil 19:6. https://doi.org/10.1186/s12984-021-00961-w

Cho J-H, Kwon B-H, Lee B-H, Lee S-W (2022) Decoding continual muscle movements related to complex hand grasping from EEG signals. In: Proceedings of the 2022 10th international winter conference on brain–computer interface (BCI). IEEE, Gangwon-do, pp 1–5

Chowdhury A, Raza H, Meena YK et al (2019) An EEG-EMG correlation-based brain–computer interface for hand orthosis supported neuro-rehabilitation. J Neurosci Methods 312:1–11. https://doi.org/10.1016/j.jneumeth.2018.11.010

Crosson B, Ford A, McGregor KM et al (2010) Functional imaging and related techniques: an introduction for rehabilitation researchers. J Rehabil Res Develop 47:7–34. https://doi.org/10.1682/JRRD.2010.02.0017

Demain S, Metcalf CD, Merrett GV et al (2013) A narrative review on haptic devices: relating the physiology and psychophysical properties of the hand to devices for rehabilitation in central nervous system disorders. Disabil Rehabil Assist Technol 8:181–189. https://doi.org/10.3109/17483107.2012.697532

Dietz V, Fouad K (2014) Restoration of sensorimotor functions after spinal cord injury. Brain 137:654–667. https://doi.org/10.1093/brain/awt262

Ding Z, Yang C, Wang Z et al (2021) Online adaptive prediction of human motion intention based on sEMG. Sensors 21:2882. https://doi.org/10.3390/s21082882

Donati ARC, Shokur S, Morya E et al (2016) Long-term training with a brain–machine interface-based gait protocol induces partial neurological recovery in paraplegic patients. Sci Rep 79:N13–N14. https://doi.org/10.1227/NEU.0000000000001451

Ethier C, Gallego JA, Miller L (2015) Brain-controlled neuromuscular stimulation to drive neural plasticity and functional recovery. Curr Opin Neurobiol 33:95–102. https://doi.org/10.1016/j.conb.2015.03.007

Fan SC, Su FC, Chen SS et al (2014) Improved intrinsic motivation and muscle activation patterns in reaching task using virtual reality training for stroke rehabilitation: a pilot randomized control trial. J Med Biol Eng 34:399–407. https://doi.org/10.5405/jmbe.1502

Feitosa JA, Fernandes CA, Casseb RF, Castellano G (2022) Effects of virtual reality-based motor rehabilitation: a systematic review of fMRI studies. J Neural Eng 19:011002. https://doi.org/10.1088/1741-2552/ac456e

Ganzer PD, Colachis SC, Schwemmer MA et al (2020) Restoring the sense of touch using a sensorimotor demultiplexing neural interface. Cell 181:763-773.e12. https://doi.org/10.1016/j.cell.2020.03.054

Gao N, Chen P, Liang L (2023) BCI–VR-based hand soft rehabilitation system with its applications in hand rehabilitation after stroke. Int J Precis Eng Manufact 24:1403–1424. https://doi.org/10.1007/s12541-023-00835-2

Gatti R, Atum Y, Schiaffino L et al (2021) Decoding kinetic features of hand motor preparation from single-trial EEG using convolutional neural networks. Eur J Neurosci 53:556–570. https://doi.org/10.1111/ejn.14936

Geng Y, Qin L, Li Y et al (2022) Identifying oscillations under multi-site sensory stimulation for high-level peripheral nerve injured patients: a pilot study. J Neural Eng 19:036028. https://doi.org/10.1088/1741-2552/ac7079

Ghassemi M, Triandafilou K, Barry A et al (2019) Development of an EMG-controlled serious game for rehabilitation. IEEE Trans Neural Syst Rehabil Eng 27:283–292. https://doi.org/10.1109/TNSRE.2019.2894102

Gómez C, Poza J, Gutiérrez MT et al (2016) Characterization of EEG patterns in brain-injured subjects and controls after a Snoezelen® intervention. Comput Methods Progr Biomed 136:1–9. https://doi.org/10.1016/j.cmpb.2016.08.008

Grosse-Wentrup M, Mattia D, Oweiss K (2011) Using brain–computer interfaces to induce neural plasticity and restore function. J Neural Eng 8:025004. https://doi.org/10.1088/1741-2560/8/2/025004

Gu Y, Xu Y, Shen Y et al (2022) A review of hand function rehabilitation systems based on hand motion recognition devices and artificial intelligence. Brain Sci 12:1079. https://doi.org/10.3390/brainsci12081079

Gulyás D, Jochumsen M (2024) Detection of movement-related brain activity associated with hand and tongue movements from single-trial around-ear EEG. Sensors 24:6004. https://doi.org/10.3390/s24186004

Guo L, Zhang B, Wang J et al (2022a) Wearable intelligent machine learning rehabilitation assessment for stroke patients compared with clinician assessment. J Clin Med 11:7467. https://doi.org/10.3390/jcm11247467

Guo CC, Chiesa PA, de Moor C et al (2022b) Digital devices for assessing motor functions in mobility-impaired and healthy populations: systematic literature review. J Med Internet Res 24:e37683. https://doi.org/10.2196/37683

Hadjiaros M, Neokleous K, Shimi A et al (2023) Virtual reality cognitive gaming based on brain computer interfacing: a narrative review. IEEE Access 11:18399–18416. https://doi.org/10.1109/ACCESS.2023.3247133

Helmer RJN, Farrow D, Ball K et al (2011) A pilot evaluation of an electronic textile for lower limb monitoring and interactive biofeedback. In: Procedia engineering, pp 513–518

Hogan N, Krebs HI, Rohrer B et al (2006) Motions or muscles? Some behavioral factors underlying robotic assistance of motor recovery. J Rehabil Res Dev 43:605–618. https://doi.org/10.1682/JRRD.2005.06.0103

Höhler C, Wild L, de Crignis A et al (2023) Contralaterally EMG-triggered functional electrical stimulation during serious gaming for upper limb stroke rehabilitation: a feasibility study. Front Neurorobot 17:1168322. https://doi.org/10.3389/fnbot.2023.1168322

Hong B, Guo F, Liu T et al (2009) N200-speller using motion-onset visual response. Clin Neurophysiol 120:1658–1666

Hu X-L, Tong RK-Y, Ho NSK et al (2015) Wrist rehabilitation assisted by an electromyography-driven neuromuscular electrical stimulation robot after stroke. Neurorehabil Neural Rep 29:767–776. https://doi.org/10.1177/1545968314565510

Hu M, Cheng H-J, Ji F et al (2021) Brain functional changes in stroke following rehabilitation using brain–computer interface-assisted motor imagery with and without tDCS: a pilot study. Front Hum Neurosci 15:692304. https://doi.org/10.3389/fnhum.2021.692304

In H, Kang BK, Sin M, Cho K (2015) Exo-glove: a soft wearable robot for the hand using soft tendon routing system. IEEE Robot Autom 22:97–105. https://doi.org/10.1109/MRA.2014.2362863

Jiang Y, Liu Z, Liu T et al (2023) A serious game system for upper limb motor function assessment of hemiparetic stroke patients. IEEE Trans Neural Syst Rehabil Eng 31:2640–2653. https://doi.org/10.1109/TNSRE.2023.3281408

Jiang YC, Zheng C, Ma R et al (2024) Within-session reliability of fNIRS in robot-assisted upper-limb training. IEEE Trans Neural Syst Rehabil Eng 32:1302–1313. https://doi.org/10.1109/TNSRE.2024.3378467

Jiang N, Dremstrup K, Farina D (2014a) A novel brain–computer interface for chronic stroke. In: Brain–computer interface research, pp 51–61

Jiang N, Mrachacz-kersting N, Xu R et al (2014b) An accurate, versatile, and robust brain switch for neurorehabilitation. In: Guger C, Vaughan T, Allison B (eds) Brain–computer interface research, 1st edn. Springer, Cham, pp 47–61

Jiang S, Chen L, Wang Z et al (2015) Application of BCI-FES system on stroke rehabilitation. In: International IEEE/EMBS conference on neural engineering, NER, pp 1112–1115

Johansson BB (2011) Current trends in stroke rehabilitation: a review with focus on brain plasticity. Acta Neurol Scand 123:147–159. https://doi.org/10.1111/j.1600-0404.2010.01417.x

Joshua AM (2022) Physiotherapy for adult neurological conditions, 1st edn. Springer, Singapore

Karimi R, Mohammadi A, Asif A, Benali H (2022) DF-SSmVEP: dual frequency aggregated steady-state motion visual evoked potential design with bifold canonical correlation analysis. Sensors 22:2568. https://doi.org/10.3390/s22072568

Kasashima Y, Fujiwara T, Matsushika Y et al (2012) Modulation of event-related desynchronization during motor imagery with transcranial direct current stimulation (tDCS) in patients with chronic hemiparetic stroke. Exp Brain Res 221:263–268. https://doi.org/10.1007/s00221-012-3166-9

Kraus D, Naros G, Bauer R et al (2016) Brain state-dependent transcranial magnetic closed-loop stimulation controlled by sensorimotor desynchronization induces robust increase of corticospinal excitability. Brain Stimul 9:415–424. https://doi.org/10.1016/j.brs.2016.02.007

Krebs HI, Palazzolo JJ, Dipietro L et al (2003) Rehabilitation robotics: performance-based progressive robot-assisted therapy. Auton Robots 15:7–20. https://doi.org/10.1023/A:1024494031121

Kwon J, Hwang J, Nam H, Im CH (2022) Novel hybrid visual stimuli incorporating periodic motions into conventional flickering or pattern-reversal visual stimuli for steady-state visual evoked potential-based brain–computer interfaces. Front Neuroinform 16:997068. https://doi.org/10.3389/fninf.2022.997068

Langhorne P, Bernhardt J, Kwakkel G (2011) Stroke rehabilitation. Lancet 377:1693–1702. https://doi.org/10.1016/S0140-6736(11)60325-5

Leamy DJ, Kocijan J, Domijan K et al (2014) An exploration of EEG features during recovery following stroke: implications for BCI-mediated neurorehabilitation therapy. J Neuroeng Rehabil 11:1–16. https://doi.org/10.1186/1743-0003-11-9

Leonardis D, Barsotti M, Loconsole C et al (2015) An EMG-controlled robotic hand exoskeleton for bilateral rehabilitation. IEEE Trans Hapt 8:140–151. https://doi.org/10.1109/TOH.2015.2417570

Levy RM, Harvey RL, Kissela BM et al (2016) Epidural electrical stimulation for stroke rehabilitation: results of the prospective, multicenter, randomized, single-blinded Everest trial. Neurorehabil Neural Repair 30:107–119. https://doi.org/10.1177/1545968315575613

Li L, Wang J, Xu G et al (2015) The study of object-oriented motor imagery based on EEG suppression. PLoS ONE 10:1–10. https://doi.org/10.1371/journal.pone.0144256

Li M, Xu G, Xie J, Chen C (2018) A review: motor rehabilitation after stroke with control based on human intent. Proc Inst Mech Eng H 232:344–360. https://doi.org/10.1177/0954411918755828

Li X, Wang L, Miao S et al (2022a) Sensorimotor rhythm-brain computer interface with audio-cue, motor observation and multisensory feedback for upper-limb stroke rehabilitation: a controlled study. Front Neurosci 16:808830. https://doi.org/10.3389/fnins.2022.808830

Li L, Zhang Y, Huang L et al (2022b) Robot assisted treatment of hand functional rehabilitation based on visual motor imagination. Front Aging Neurosci 14:870871. https://doi.org/10.3389/fnagi.2022.870871

Li N, Yang Y, Li G et al (2024) Multi-sensor fusion-based mirror adaptive assist-as-needed control strategy of a soft exoskeleton for upper limb rehabilitation. IEEE Trans Autom Sci Eng 21:475–487. https://doi.org/10.1109/TASE.2022.3225727

Liang S, Choi K-S, Qin J et al (2016) Improving the discrimination of hand motor imagery via virtual reality based visual guidance. Comput Methods Progr Biomed 132:63–74. https://doi.org/10.1016/j.cmpb.2016.04.023

Lorenz EA, Su X, Skjæret-Maroni N (2024) A review of combined functional neuroimaging and motion capture for motor rehabilitation. J Neuroeng Rehabil 21:3. https://doi.org/10.1186/s12984-023-01294-6

Lu C, Ge R, Tang Z et al (2023) Multi-channel FES gait rehabilitation assistance system based on adaptive sEMG modulation. IEEE Trans Neural Syst Rehabil Eng 31:3652–3663. https://doi.org/10.1109/TNSRE.2023.3313617

Luo W, Yin W, Liu Q, Qu Y (2023) A hybrid brain–computer interface using motor imagery and SSVEP based on convolutional neural network. Brain Apparat Commun J Bacom 2:2258938. https://doi.org/10.1080/27706710.2023.2258938

Lyukmanov RKh, Isaev MR, Mokienko OA et al (2024) Brain–computer interface using functional near-infrared spectroscopy for post-stroke motor rehabilitation: case series. Ann Clin Exper Neurol 17:82–88

Macdonell RAL, Donnan GA, Bladin PF (1989) A comparison of somatosensory evoked and motor evoked potentials in stroke. Ann Neurol 25:68–73. https://doi.org/10.1002/ana.410250111

Magistris MR, Rösler KM, Truffert A, Myers JP (1998) Transcranial stimulation excites virtually all motor neurons supplying the target muscle: a demonstration and a method improving the study of motor evoked potentials. Brain 121:437–450. https://doi.org/10.1093/brain/121.3.437

Marchal-Crespo L, Reinkensmeyer DJ (2009) Review of control strategies for robotic movement training after neurologic injury. J Neuroeng Rehabil 6:20. https://doi.org/10.1186/1743-0003-6-20

Moxon KA, Oliviero A, Aguilar J, Foffani G (2014) Cortical reorganization after spinal cord injury: always for good? Neuroscience 283:78–94. https://doi.org/10.1016/j.neuroscience.2014.06.056

Mrachacz-Kersting N, Kristensen SR, Niazi IK, Farina D (2012) Precise temporal association between cortical potentials evoked by motor imagination and afference induces cortical plasticity. J Physiol 590:1669–1682. https://doi.org/10.1113/jphysiol.2011.222851

Niazi IK, Mrachacz-Kersting N, Jiang N et al (2012) Peripheral electrical stimulation triggered by self-paced detection of motor intention enhances motor evoked potentials. IEEE Trans Neural Syst Rehabil Eng 20:595–604. https://doi.org/10.1109/TNSRE.2012.2194309

Nicolas-Alonso LF, Gomez-Gil J (2012) Brain computer interfaces, a review. Sensors 12:1211–1279. https://doi.org/10.3390/s120201211

Nitsche MA, Paulus W (2000) Excitability changes induced in the human motor cortex by weak transcranial direct current stimulation. J Physiol 527(3):633–639

Nojima I, Sugata H, Takeuchi H, Mima T (2022) Brain–computer interface training based on brain activity can induce motor recovery in patients with stroke: a meta-analysis. Neurorehabil Neural Repair 36:83–96. https://doi.org/10.1177/15459683211062895

Norman SL, Wolpaw JR, Reinkensmeyer DJ (2022) Targeting neuroplasticity to improve motor recovery after stroke: an artificial neural network model. Brain Commun 4:fcac264. https://doi.org/10.1093/braincomms/fcac264

Norris TA, Augenstein TE, Rodriguez KM et al (2024) Shaping corticospinal pathways in virtual reality: effects of task complexity and sensory feedback during mirror therapy in neurologically intact individuals. J Neuroeng Rehabil 21:154. https://doi.org/10.1186/s12984-024-01454-2

Ono T, Mukaino M, Ushiba J (2013) Functional recovery in upper limb function in stroke survivors by using brain–computer interface A single case A–B–A–B design. Conf Proc IEEE Eng Med Biol Soc 2013:265–268. https://doi.org/10.1109/EMBC.2013.6609488

Ortega P, Faisal AA (2021) Deep learning multimodal fNIRS and EEG signals for bimanual grip force decoding. J Neural Eng 18:0460e6

Özgünen KT, Çelik U, Kurdak SS (2010) Determination of an optimal threshold value for muscle activity detection in EMG analysis. J Sports Sci Med 9:620

Oztop E, Kawato M, Arbib MA (2013) Mirror neurons: functions, mechanisms and models. Neurosci Lett 540:43–55. https://doi.org/10.1016/j.neulet.2012.10.005

Ozturk A, Tartar A, Ersoz Huseyinsinoglu B, Ertas AH (2016) A clinically feasible kinematic assessment method of upper extremity motor function impairment after stroke. Measurement 80:207–216

Park EC, Hwangbo G (2015) The effects of action observation gait training on the static balance and walking ability of stroke patients. J Phys Ther Sci 27:341–344. https://doi.org/10.1589/jpts.27.341

Pascual-Leone A, Freitas C, Oberman L et al (2011) Characterizing brain cortical plasticity and network dynamics across the age-span in health and disease with TMS-EEG and TMS-fMRI. Brain Topogr 24:302–315. https://doi.org/10.1007/s10548-011-0196-8

Patel J, Fluet G, Merians A et al (2015) Virtual reality-augmented rehabilitation in the acute phase post-stroke for individuals with flaccid upper extremities: a feasibility study. In: Proceedings of the 2015 international conference on virtual rehabilitation (ICVR), pp 215–223

Pfurtscheller G (2010) The hybrid BCI. Front Neurosci 4:1–11. https://doi.org/10.3389/fnpro.2010.00003

Pichiorri F, Morone G, Petti M et al (2015) Brain–computer interface boosts motor imagery practice during stroke recovery. Ann Neurol 77:851–865. https://doi.org/10.1002/ana.24390

Piggott L, Wagner S, Ziat M (2016) Haptic neurorehabilitation and virtual reality for upper limb paralysis: a review. Crit Rev Biomed Eng 1–2:1–32. https://doi.org/10.1615/CritRevBiomedEng.2016016046

Porciuncula F, Roto AV, Kumar D et al (2018) Wearable movement sensors for rehabilitation: a focused review of technological and clinical advances. PMR 10:S220–S232. https://doi.org/10.1016/j.pmrj.2018.06.013

Proulx CE, Louis Jean MT, Higgins J et al (2022) Somesthetic, visual, and auditory feedback and their interactions applied to upper limb neurorehabilitation technology: a narrative review to facilitate contextualization of knowledge. Front Rehabil Sci 3:789479. https://doi.org/10.3389/fresc.2022.789479

Quandt F, Hummel FC (2014) The influence of functional electrical stimulation on hand motor recovery in stroke patients: a review. Exp Transl Stroke Med 6:9. https://doi.org/10.1186/2040-7378-6-9

Ramos-Murguialday A, Broetz D, Rea M et al (2013) Brain–machine interface in chronic stroke rehabilitation: a controlled study. Ann Neurol 74:100–108. https://doi.org/10.1002/ana.23879

Ranzani R, Lambercy O, Metzger JC et al (2020) Neurocognitive robot-assisted rehabilitation of hand function: a randomized control trial on motor recovery in subacute stroke. J Neuroeng Rehabil 17:1–13. https://doi.org/10.1186/s12984-020-00746-7

Remsik AB, van Kan PLE, Gloe S et al (2022) BCI-FES with multimodal feedback for motor recovery poststroke. Front Hum Neurosci 16:725715. https://doi.org/10.3389/fnhum.2022.725715

Resquín F, Cuesta Gomez A, Gonzalez-Vargas J et al (2016) Hybrid robotic systems for upper limb rehabilitation after stroke: a review. Med Eng Phys 38:1279–1288. https://doi.org/10.1016/j.medengphy.2016.09.001

Ricciardi E, Vanello N, Sani L et al (2007) The effect of visual experience on the development of functional architecture in hMT+. Cereb Cortex 17:2933–2939. https://doi.org/10.1093/cercor/bhm018

Rojas-Martínez M, Serna LY, Jordanic M et al (2020) High-density surface electromyography signals during isometric contractions of elbow muscles of healthy humans. Sci Data 7:397. https://doi.org/10.1038/s41597-020-00717-6

Rossi S, Hallett M, Rossini PM, Pascual-Leone A (2009) Safety, ethical considerations, and application guidelines for the use of transcranial magnetic stimulation in clinical practice and research. Clin Neurophysiol 120:2008–2039. https://doi.org/10.1016/j.clinph.2009.08.016

Said RR, Bin HMB, Song K et al (2022) A systematic review of virtual reality and robot therapy as recent rehabilitation technologies using EEG-brain–computer interface based on movement-related cortical potentials. Biosensors 12:1134. https://doi.org/10.3390/bios12121134

Saposnik G (2016) Virtual reality in stroke rehabilitation. In: Ovbiagele B (ed) Ischemic stroke therapeutics. Springer, Cham, pp 225–233

Scotto di Luzio F, Cordella F, Bravi M et al (2022) Modification of hand muscular synergies in stroke patients after robot-aided rehabilitation. Appl Sci 12:3146. https://doi.org/10.3390/app12063146

Secoli R, Milot M-H, Rosati G, Reinkensmeyer DJ (2011) Effect of visual distraction and auditory feedback on patient effort during robot-assisted movement training after stroke. J Neuroeng Rehabil 8:21. https://doi.org/10.1186/1743-0003-8-21

Semprini M, Cuppone A, Squeri V, Konczak J (2015) Muscle innervation patterns for human wrist control: useful biofeedback signals for robotic rehabilitation? IEEE international conference on rehabilitation robotics. IEEE, Singapore, pp 919–924

Sharma N, Upadhyay A, Sharma M, Singhal A (2023) Deep temporal networks for EEG-based motor imagery recognition. Sci Rep 13:18813. https://doi.org/10.1038/s41598-023-41653-w

Shi Y, Shen G (2024) Haptic sensing and feedback techniques toward virtual reality. Research 7:0333

Sigrist R, Rauter G, Riener R, Wolf P (2013) Augmented visual, auditory, haptic, and multimodal feedback in motor learning: a review. Psychon Bull Rev 20:21–53. https://doi.org/10.3758/s13423-012-0333-8

Solo-Faraco S, Spence C, Lloyd D, Kingstone A (2004) Moving multisensory research along: motion perception across sensory modalities. Curr Dir Psychol Sci 13:29–32. https://doi.org/10.1111/j.0963-7214.2004.01301008.x

Song R, Tong K-Y, Hu X, Zhou W (2013a) Myoelectrically controlled wrist robot for stroke rehabilitation. J Neuroeng Rehabil 10:52. https://doi.org/10.1186/1743-0003-10-52

Song R, Tong KY, Hu X et al (2013b) Arm-eye coordination test to objectively quantify motor performance and muscles activation in persons after stroke undergoing robot-aided rehabilitation training: a pilot study. Exp Brain Res 229:373–382. https://doi.org/10.1007/s00221-013-3418-3

Su W-C, Dashtestani H, Miguel HO et al (2023) Simultaneous multimodal fNIRS-EEG recordings reveal new insights in neural activity during motor execution, observation, and imagery. Sci Rep 13:5151. https://doi.org/10.1038/s41598-023-31609-5

Su J, Wang J, Wang W et al (2024) Enhanced motor imagery based brain–computer interface via vibration stimulation and robotic glove for post-stroke rehabilitation. In: Communications in computer and information science, pp 326–337

Sun R, Song R, Tong K (2014) Complexity analysis of EMG signals for patients after stroke during robot-aided rehabilitation training using fuzzy approximate entropy. IEEE Trans Neural Syst Rehabil Eng 22:1013–1019. https://doi.org/10.1109/TNSRE.2013.2290017

Sun X, Dai C, Wu X et al (2024) Current implications of EEG and fNIRS as functional neuroimaging techniques for motor recovery after stroke. Med Rev 4:492–509. https://doi.org/10.1515/mr-2024-0010

Swarnakar R, Yadav SL (2023) Artificial intelligence and machine learning in motor recovery: a rehabilitation medicine perspective. World J Clin Cases 11:7258–7260

Takeuchi N, Izumi S-I (2013) Rehabilitation with poststroke motor recovery: a review with a focus on neural plasticity. Stroke Res Treat 2013:128641. https://doi.org/10.1155/2013/128641

Tang C, Zhou T, Zhang Y et al (2023) Bilateral upper limb robot-assisted rehabilitation improves upper limb motor function in stroke patients: a study based on quantitative EEG. Eur J Med Res 28:603. https://doi.org/10.1186/s40001-023-01565-x

Teo WP, Chew E (2014) Is motor-imagery brain–computer interface feasible in stroke rehabilitation? PMR 6:723–728. https://doi.org/10.1016/j.pmrj.2014.01.006

Thøgersen M, Hansen J, Arendt-Nielsen L et al (2018) Removing own-limb visual input using mixed reality (MR) produces a "telescoping" illusion in healthy individuals. Behav Brain Res 347:263. https://doi.org/10.1016/j.bbr.2018.03.024

Turolla A, Daud Albasini OA, Oboe R et al (2013) Haptic-based neurorehabilitation in poststroke patients: a feasibility prospective multicentre trial for robotics hand rehabilitation. Comput Math Methods Med 2013:895492. https://doi.org/10.1155/2013/895492

Umeda T, Isa T, Nishimura Y (2019) The somatosensory cortex receives information about motor output. Sci Adv 5:eaaw5388. https://doi.org/10.1126/sciadv.aaw5388

van Dokkum LEH, Ward T, Laffont I (2015) Brain computer interfaces for neurorehabilitation-its current status as a rehabilitation strategy post-stroke. Ann Phys Rehabil Med 58:3–8. https://doi.org/10.1016/j.rehab.2014.09.016

Vansteensel MJ, Pels EGM, Bleichner MG et al (2016) Fully implanted brain–computer interface in a locked-in patient with ALS. N Engl J Med 375:2060–2066

Várkuti B, Guan C, Pan Y et al (2013) Resting state changes in functional connectivity correlate with movement recovery for BCI and robot-assisted upper-extremity training after stroke. Neurorehabil Neural Rep 27:53–62. https://doi.org/10.1177/1545968312445910

Vuckovic A, Osuagwu BA (2013) Using a motor imagery questionnaire to estimate the performance of a brain–computer interface based on object oriented motor imagery. Clin Neurophysiol 124:1586–1595. https://doi.org/10.1016/j.clinph.2013.02.016

Wade E, Winstein CJ (2012) Virtual reality and robotics for stroke rehabilitation: where do we go from here? Top Stroke Rehabil 18:685–700. https://doi.org/10.1310/tsr1806-685

Wahl T, Riedinger J, Duprez M, Hutt A (2023) Delayed closed-loop neurostimulation for the treatment of pathological brain rhythms in mental disorders: a computational study. Front Neurosci 17:1183670. https://doi.org/10.3389/fnins.2023.1183670

Warraich Z, Kleim JA (2010) Neural plasticity: the biological substrate for neurorehabilitation. PMR 2:S208–S219. https://doi.org/10.1016/j.pmrj.2010.10.016

Wieloch T, Nikolich K (2006) Mechanisms of neural plasticity following brain injury. Curr Opin Neurobiol 16:258–264. https://doi.org/10.1016/j.conb.2006.05.011

Wolpaw JR, Birbaumer N, McFarland DJ et al (2002) Brain–computer interfaces for communication and control. Clin Neurophysiol 113:767–791. https://doi.org/10.1016/S1388-2457(02)00057-3

Wolters A, Sandbrink F, Schlottmann A et al (2003) A temporally asymmetric Hebbian rule governing plasticity in the human motor cortex. J Neurophysiol 89:2339–2345. https://doi.org/10.1152/jn.00900.2002

World Health Organization (2020) The top 10 causes of death—factsheet

Wright ZA, Rymer WZ, Slutzky MW (2014) Reducing abnormal muscle coactivation after stroke using a myoelectric-computer interface: a pilot study. Neurorehabil Neural Repair 28:443–451. https://doi.org/10.1177/1545968313517751

Wurzinger H, Abzhandadze T, Rafsten L, Sunnerhagen KS (2021) Dependency in activities of daily living during the first year after stroke. Front Neurol 12:736684. https://doi.org/10.3389/fneur.2021.736684

Xie J, Xu G, Wang J et al (2012) Steady-state motion visual evoked potentials produced by oscillating Newton's rings: implications for brain–computer interfaces. PLoS ONE 7:e39707. https://doi.org/10.1371/journal.pone.0039707

Xu R, Jiang N, Lin C et al (2014) Enhanced low-latency detection of motor intention from EEG for closed-loop brain–computer interface applications. IEEE Trans Biomed Eng 61:288–296. https://doi.org/10.1109/TBME.2013.2294203

Xu Y, McClelland VM, Cvetkovic Z, Mills KR (2016) Corticomuscular coherence with time lag with application to delay estimation. IEEE Trans Biomed Eng 64:1–600. https://doi.org/10.1109/TBME.2016.2569492

Yan W, Xu G, Li M et al (2017) Steady-state motion visual evoked potential (SSMVEP) based on equal luminance colored enhancement. PLoS ONE 12:e0169642. https://doi.org/10.1371/journal.pone.0169642

Yang S, Li M, Wang J et al (2023) A low-cost and portable wrist exoskeleton using EEG-sEMG combined strategy for prolonged active rehabilitation. Front Neurorobot 17:1161187. https://doi.org/10.3389/fnbot.2023.1161187

Yilmaz O, Birbaumer N, Ramos-Murguialday A (2015) Movement related slow cortical potentials in severely paralyzed chronic stroke patients. Front Hum Neurosci 8:1033. https://doi.org/10.3389/fnhum.2014.01033

Yu Y, Chen Y, Lou T, Shen X (2022) Correlation between proprioceptive impairment and motor deficits after stroke: a meta-analysis review. Front Neurol 12:688616. https://doi.org/10.3389/fneur.2021.688616

Zbytniewska M, Kanzler CM, Jordan L et al (2021) Reliable and valid robot-assisted assessments of hand proprioceptive, motor and sensorimotor impairments after stroke. J Neuroeng Rehabil 18:115. https://doi.org/10.1186/s12984-021-00904-5

Zhang J, Wang B, Zhang C et al (2019) An EEG/EMG/EOG-based multimodal human-machine interface to real-time control of a soft robot hand. Front Neurorobot 13:00007. https://doi.org/10.3389/fnbot.2019.00007

Zhang X, Hou W, Wu X et al (2021) A novel online action observation-based brain–computer interface that enhances event-related desynchronization. IEEE Trans Neural Syst Rehabil Eng 29:2605–2614. https://doi.org/10.1109/TNSRE.2021.3133853

Zhang J, Liu D, Chen W et al (2022) Deep convolutional neural network for EEG-based motor decoding. Micromachines 13:1485. https://doi.org/10.3390/mi13091485

Zheng J, Ma Q, He W et al (2023) Cognitive and motor cortex activation during robot-assisted multi-sensory interactive motor rehabilitation training: an fNIRS based pilot study. Front Hum Neurosci 17:1089276. https://doi.org/10.3389/fnhum.2023.1089276

Zschorlich VR, Behrendt F, de Lussanet MHE (2021) Multimodal sensorimotor integration of visual and kinaesthetic afferents modulates motor circuits in humans. Brain Sci 11:187. https://doi.org/10.3390/brainsci11020187

Zulauf-Czaja A, Al-Taleb MKH, Purcell M et al (2021) On the way home: a BCI-FES hand therapy self-managed by sub-acute SCI participants and their caregivers: a usability study. J Neuroeng Rehabil 18:44. https://doi.org/10.1186/s12984-021-00838-y

Chapter 2
Revolutionizing Hand Rehabilitation: Soft Wearable Hand Robots

Wearable hand robots are designed to be directly attached to human hands, supporting and augmenting locomotor capacity for a broad spectrum of rehabilitative and assistive applications. Recent advancements emphasize the use of soft hand exoskeletons, addressing joint misalignment issues while improving safety and comfort. This chapter explores user needs and technological requirements for soft wearable hand robots in rehabilitation, assistance, and haptic feedback applications. It evaluates recent innovations in mechanism design, motion monitoring, force detection, and control methods. Furthermore, it introduces a novel soft robotic glove designed for finger abduction support, offering enhanced assistance for complex hand motions compared to current devices.

2.1 Introduction

The human hand's complex anatomy—comprising 27 bones, 16 joints, and 22 degrees of freedom (DOFs)—makes it highly functional yet vulnerable to various impairments (Dai et al. 2009). Conditions like stroke-induced hemiparesis, injuries, and degenerative diseases can severely affect hand functionality, limiting the ability to perform Activities of Daily Living (ADLs), and thus diminishing overall quality of life (Heo et al. 2012). Research on robot-assisted wrist and hand training has demonstrated that functional impairments in the distal joints can influence the overall function of the arm (Lambercy et al. 2011). The neurological disorder known as "finger muscle weakness", particularly relevant to extensor muscles, is regarded as a key contributor to hand dysfunction following a stroke (Kamper et al. 2006). It is important to note that approximately 30–40% of stroke survivors typically experience hypertonia (Thibaut et al. 2013). This condition is characterized by abnormally elevated muscle tension caused by impairment to the central nervous system. Moreover, for people working in heavy industry, military, construction, nursing home,

M. Li and B. He, *Intention-Controlled Hand Rehabilitation for Stroke Survivors*,
https://doi.org/10.1007/978-981-95-4196-6_2

and logistics, augmenting the hand function, in terms of amplifying the applied force or automating the motion, is often required to help the operator handle heavier loads or over longer periods of time (Heo et al. 2012). The advent of an aging society, and the increasing demand for practical applications of hand rehabilitation and assistance, indicate the need for portable solutions that can be integrated into everyday living outside of the context of rehabilitation clinics. In virtual reality applications, the integration of portable haptic devices designed for body-worn use is also desired to create a more immersive experience in virtual world interaction. Moreover, in extreme environments such as nuclear reactors, space and offshore missions as well as post-earthquake and fire scenarios, a wearable hand robot can enhance safety and dexterity of manipulation. Wearable hand robots, often referred as hand exoskeletons, are comprised of actuation and sensing mechanisms supporting and augmenting users' hand movements. This class of robots are particularly useful for repetitive training of hand muscles for rehabilitation, assistance in daily tasks, haptic feedback, or tele-manipulation applications.

The rigid mechanical design of linkage-based (Chiri et al. 2012) and rack-and-pinion mechanisms (Worsnopp et al. 2007) provides a robust and reliable means of power transmission in various rehabilitation or human augmentation scenarios (Sandoval-gonzalez et al. 2016; Jo and Bae 2017; Bianchi et al. 2018), including hand exoskeleton devices (Ito et al. 2011; Cui et al. 2015). However, the linkage structure requires a rotation center aligned with the respective axis of rotation in human finger joint (Heo et al. 2012). Even if the joints of robot and human finger are initially aligned in one position, a misalignment of the joints may occur during rehabilitation movements which requires compensation (Cui et al. 2015) (see Fig. 2.1a). Current compensation approaches inevitably increase the complexity of the linkage mechanism (Fang et al. 2009; Ho et al. 2011). Moreover, the rigid mechanical design can lead to users' discomfort or induce health and safety issues. Therefore, an experienced oversee is required when these robotic devices are in use (Polygerinos et al. 2015a). In addition, the bulky and complex rigid linkage structure makes hand exoskeleton devices cumbersome (Arata et al. 2013) (see Fig. 2.1). The aforementioned drawbacks hinder practical applications of this conventional type of exoskeletons.

In recent years, there is a trend towards soft wearable mechanisms that dispense with rigid frames for hand exoskeleton. Using these soft wearable mechanisms avoids joint misalignment problems. For mechanisms where flexible, jointless structures

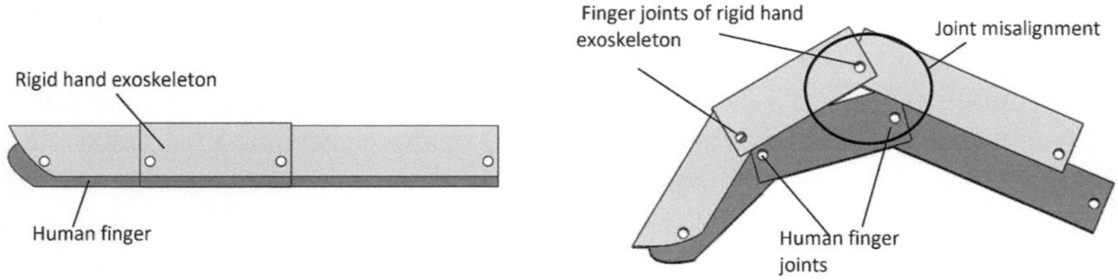

Fig. 2.1 Rigid wearable hand robots suffering from the joint misalignment problem

have been utilized, the user's hand provides skeletal structures for the robot motion (Heo et al. 2012). Moreover, soft wearable hand robots usually need less space and are lighter than their rigid equivalents. Terms such as "exoglove" (Yap et al. 2015a), "wearable soft robotic glove" (Radder et al. 2020), and "jointless tendon-driven hand exoskeleton" (Yang et al. 2016) have all been used to describe soft hand robots.

A narrative review by Chu and Patterson (2018) highlighted soft robotic systems designed for hand rehabilitation and support, examining aspects like portability, safety, and feedback inputs. However, recent advancements in soft robotics have expanded their applications beyond rehabilitation to include haptic feedback and improved control algorithms. This chapter provides a comprehensive review of these advancements and discusses the user requirements for soft wearable hand robots across rehabilitation, assistance, and haptic feedback applications.

Then, we describe the development and manufacturing process of two types of pneumatically actuated soft hand exoskeletons, 3D printed from flexible materials, featuring assisted finger abduction and independent flexion control of individual finger joints. Compared to existing hand exoskeletons, the devices can provide assistance to finger abduction movements and enable independent control of finger joint motions, thereby offering more effective support for intricate hand movements during rehabilitation. This part in this chapter builds upon our earlier IEEE conference publications (Li et al. 2019, 2020), expanding the analysis and comparison of the two soft glove designs. While the original works focused on the design and validation of individual prototypes, this chapter provides a direct comparison, integrates additional analytical results, and presents the findings in a new format for clarity and completeness.

2.2 Applications for Soft Wearable Hand Robots

There applications of soft wearable hand robots can be classified into three main categories including rehabilitation, assistance, and haptic feedback (Perry et al. 2007). In each application, there are different user and technical requirements for the wearable hand robots.

General User Requirements for Wearable Hand Robots

It is clear that one of the most important requirements for the wearable hand robots is safety (Heo et al. 2012). To meet safety requirements, restrictions to the range of motion (ROM) should be set for the wearable hand robots to prevent hyperextension of the patient's joints; the range is conservatively set to be shorter than that of healthy people. Also, the applied external forces causing a joint movement should not exceed respective physiological values and should strictly respect the DOFs of body joints (Borboni et al. 2016). The wearable hand robots should have a certain amount of compliance so that the robot cannot hurt the subject in the case of motion trajectory errors.

A wearable hand robot should produce minimal resistance to the natural movement of fingers. Movements of the wearable hand robot should be in conformity to human hand motion patterns. Therefore, the strategies and patterns of fingers' motion should be investigated and considered in control of wearable hand robots (Vaz et al. 2017). Moreover, reduction in the weight and improvements in portability are also needed for practical use (Nycz et al. 2016).

Low complexity, compactness, smoothness and sterilizability are among other important factors in the hand exoskeleton design process. Also, the wearable hand robot should be simple to use and the user should feel psychologically comfortable about wearing it. Finally, the design should permit customization to accommodate different hand sizes and be adaptable to various hand gestures.

Soft Wearable Hand Robots for Rehabilitation Applications

It is shown that motor recovery can be greatly influenced by the post-stroke sensorimotor training (Heo et al. 2012), providing insight into possible approaches for reproducing the feeling of normal movements in patients with motion disorder and ideally, movement recovery (Reinkensmeyer et al. 2004).

The human hand contains 15 joints in total. The thumb features three joints: the interphalangeal (IP) joint, the metacarpophalangeal (MCP) joint, and the carpometacarpal (CMC) joint. Each of the other four fingers has three joints—the distal interphalangeal (DIP) joint, the proximal interphalangeal (PIP) joint, and the metacarpophalangeal (MCP) joint. For rehabilitation applications, the hand exoskeleton should feature three bending DOFs to effectively train the three joints of a human finger. Bi-directional actuation is desired to enable precise recovery from an extended or flexed configuration. For the thumb finger, an extra rotational DOF is required to match the similar ability in human thumb. Since most manual tasks do not require fingers to flex or extend to their flexion or extension extremes, designing a hand exoskeleton that can reach the entire workspace has relatively little functional relevance. The independent movements of a single-finger and several modes of multi-finger coordinated movements, for example tripod grasping, are often achievable by soft wearable rehabilitation robots. Since there are some motor synergies between fingers and finger joints, for example, the bending angles of DIP and PIP joints are related in grasping movements, it is not necessary for each of the DIP, PIP, and MCP joints of the finger to have independent movement, provided that the full ROM of the finger can be achieved for some rehabilitation applications. For example, tripod grasping requires DIP, PIP, and MCP joints of the index finger to flex ~12°, 48°, and 46°, respectively (In et al. 2015).

A wearable hand robot for hand rehabilitation should be able to generate adequate force to support and augment hand flexion and extension to enable following the movement pattern of a natural finger. Current devices can deliver a maximum output force from a single actuator ranging from 1.21 to 70.4 N (Polygerinos et al. 2013; Yap et al. 2016a). Moreover, physiotherapists suggest a minimum execution time of around 20 s for the rehabilitation exercise of finger joint in a complete flexion–extension cycle (Borboni et al. 2016).

The hand exoskeleton should be able to support the most commonly reported treatment approaches including assisted passive finger movements, assisted active finger movements, as well as resisted active finger movements (Prange et al. 2006). For assisted passive finger movements, continuous passive motion (CPM), a therapeutic approach that makes a human joint move following a predetermined sequence without any active action by the patient, has proven to effectively support the restoration of joint function for neurological patients (Winter et al. 2011). This approach does not require a highly accurate measurement of finger movements (Borboni et al. 2016). While in resisted active finger movements, the use of sensors is not mandatory (Heo et al. 2012), rehabilitation with assisted active finger movement requires sensing of finger movement and acquiring the user's motor intent; the motion data from individual joints should be provided for robust control. Beyond that, to provide a precise evaluation reference to rehabilitation therapists, the performance of the patients in conducting rehabilitation exercises should be measured and recorded during rehabilitation by integrating appropriate sensory systems.

Reduction in the weight and improvements in portability are essential for practical use of hand exoskeletons by a wider stroke population especially for in-home therapy (Nycz et al. 2016). For stroke survivors, when the load on the upper lime is increased, the abnormal synergies and weakness in elbow and shoulder joints affect active arm movements and its ROM (Beer et al. 2007). Although the amount of weight bearable by a patient is highly patient-specific and a definitive value is difficult to determine (Nycz et al. 2016), a weight of approximately 400–500 g on the hand is generally considered acceptable (Gasser and Goldfarb 2015; Aubin et al. 2014).

Soft Wearable Hand Robots for Assistive Applications

Despite undergoing intensive treatment and rehabilitation, stroke patients may still experience incomplete recovery of hand function (Go et al. 2014); 50% of stroke survivors have retained some degree of hemiparesis when measured six months after stroke (Go et al. 2014). Soft wearable hand robots can assist disabled people who have permanently lost or have significantly weakened hand function in carrying out daily tasks. They can also help able-bodied people by reducing the physical burden and augmenting their abilities. In heavy industry, military, construction, nursing home, and logistics requiring the performance of forceful and repetitive hand movements, soft wearable hand robots can be used to enhance hand function by augmenting the applied force to help the operators to carry heavier loads or to increase their strength and endurance (Heo et al. 2012). They can free people from the hard physical labor and potentially prevent work-related musculoskeletal disorders.

Additionally, the output force should assist the user in generating the necessary grasping forces to handle objects encountered in ADLs. Matheus and Dollar (2010) found that everyday objects typically weigh <1.5 kg. Polygerinos et al. (2015a) estimated that a palmar grasp, used to lift objects weighing <1.5 kg, requires an approximate fingertip force of 7.3 N, with the four fingers pressing against the palm to generate the necessary grip. Smaby et al. (2004) identified the pinch forces needed to handle or manipulate objects in ADL are typically below 20 N.

During the robotic assisting process, the motion of exoskeletons and assistive robots are expected to be in accordance with human motion to provide effective assistance and to avoid injury. Therefore, the robots should be equipped with appropriate sensors to acquire user's motor intent and measure fingers' movement. Moreover, the required output forces should be calculated according to the assistive applications.

Soft Wearable Hand Robots for Haptic Feedback Applications

In virtual reality applications, wearable haptic feedback devices are desired to increase the sense of immersion experienced during interaction with the virtual environment. In this type of applications, the forces generated by the hand robot can enable physical interaction with virtual objects; the user can convey the shape, texture, stiffness, or other characteristics of the virtual objects. Soft wearable hand robots for haptic feedback should be capable of measuring the finger's movements and presenting the reaction force to the operator (Jo and Bae 2017). The force feedback resists the user's movement and is designed to convey information about the weight, softness, and inertia of virtual objects (Bouzit et al. 2002). The inclusion of tactile feedback, force feedback, or a combination of the two, can make the interactions with virtual objects more realistic. Force feedback should be applied to known locations on the hand and fingertips. To achieve this, haptic feedback actuators for fingertips (Li et al. 2014a, b), finger pads, or palm can be added to wearable hand robots to create tactile sensation and the parameters such as positions and angles of fingertips need to be monitored.

Dexterous tele-manipulations are needed in extreme environments including fire sites, nuclear reactors, offshore infrastructure, elevated structures as well as in space (Koyama et al. 2002), where an operator would exploit advantages of a master wearable hand robot to control a slave robot in a teleoperation mode. In the case of applying wearable hand robots to a tele-manipulation system, the system should be capable of capturing the motion of the remotely operated manipulation arm (the pose of the arm) and the external forces applied to the arm at the slave side, and reflect this information back to the user's hand at the master side. Haptic feedback should also be provided to achieve better control.

It is interesting to note that most sophisticated soft wearable hand robots have been designed for power-assistance or rehabilitation applications. Only a few soft wearable hand robots [for example, Connelly et al. (2010), Ryu et al. (2008), and Zhang et al. (2018)] have been used for haptic feedback and teleoperation. Soft wearable hand robots for haptic feedback and teleoperation may be a neglected area that has a great potential for future studies.

2.3 Mechanisms of Soft Wearable Hand Robots

There are a number of distinct actuation mechanisms used in the development of soft wearable hand robots spanning from pneumatically-driven to tendon-driven, electro-active polymers and other mechanisms. It should be highlighted that in soft wearable hand robots, the actuation system for driving tendons and pneumatic or hydraulic systems can be positioned remotely to allow light-weight design of the robot. In this study, we classify the actuation mechanisms employed in soft wearable hand robots into three main categories: pneumatic or hydraulic mechanisms, tendon-driven mechanisms, and other mechanisms.

Pneumatic or Hydraulic Mechanisms

Soft robots are primarily composed of soft materials (with elasticity moduli 10^4–10^9) (Rus and Tolley 2015). Soft and elastic materials absorb mechanical stress thereby the use of these type of materials in robots makes them safer to interact with human, and potentially more crash resilient (Lee et al. 2017).

Pneumatic and hydraulic-driven soft hand exosuits, which are mainly fabricated using silicone rubber, are proposed to support finger flexion or extension (Polygerinos et al. 2015a; Yap et al. 2015a). By appropriately designing chambers, pneumatic and hydraulic actuation can deform soft bodies of the robots in a controlled way (Laschi et al. 2016). For example, simple polyurethane air tubes were used in PneuGlove, a wearable soft hand robot, to assist the hand opening (Connelly et al. 2010). Two commonly used mechanisms shown in Fig. 2.2b and 2.2c include an elastomeric tube in a woven fiber shell (Polygerinos et al. 2015a; Wang et al. 2017a) and an elastomeric tube with different cross-sections at different locations (Polygerinos et al. 2013; Yap et al. 2015b). They often contain a strain-limited layer at the one side of the tube. The tube undergoes an elongation and bends towards the strain-limited layer, when enough air pressure is applied. The latter category can be further divided into two types including an elastomeric tube containing several channel cells used in Polygerinos et al. (2013) and an elastomeric tube with varied wall thickness (Yap et al. 2015a). A limited number of studies have utilized sub-atmospheric pressure to induce contraction, buckling, or twisting motions in other soft robots (Wakimoto et al. 2009) which has not yet been applied to wearable hand robots but shows a good potential. Textile actuators (Ramos et al. 2022; Nassour et al. 2020; Cappello et al. 2018a; Maldonado-Mejía et al. 2023; Hernandez-Barraza et al. 2023; Suulker et al. 2022) can also be employed to create pneumatic or hydraulic soft wearable hand robots, offering a more compact, lightweight, and cost-effective solution.

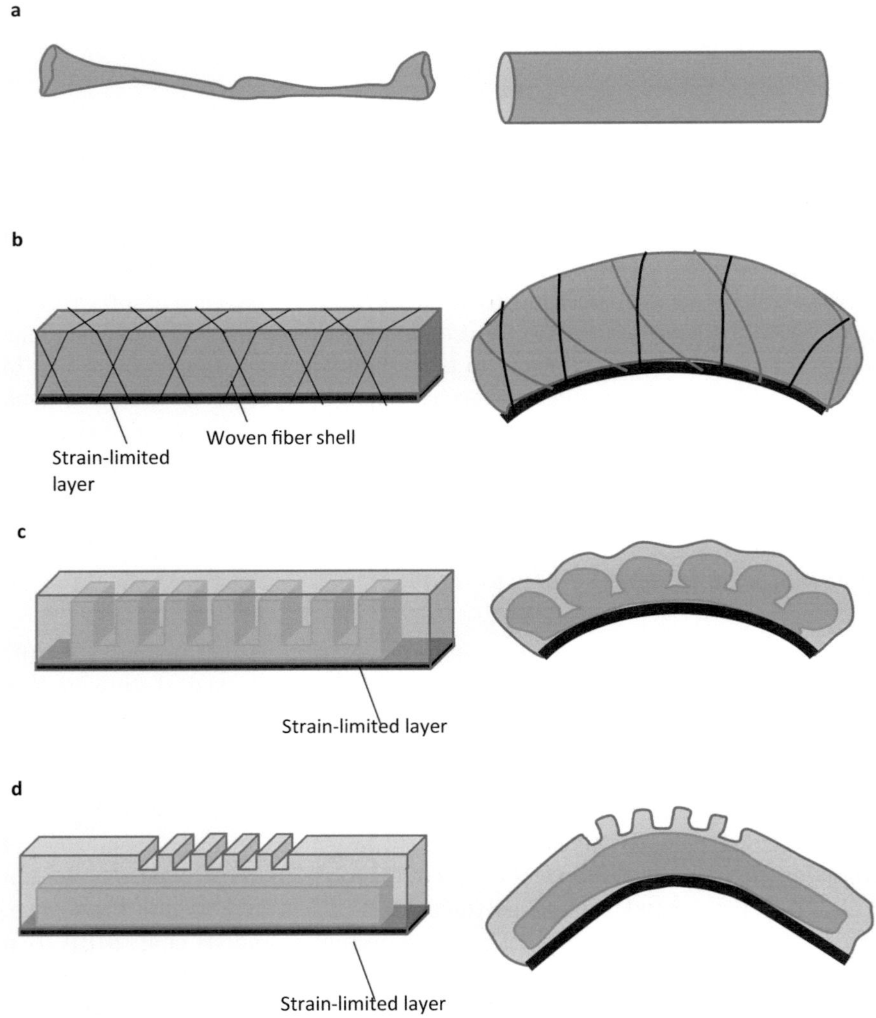

Fig. 2.2 Mechanisms for wearable soft hand robots in resting (left) and actuated (right) states: **a** simple plastic tube used in Connelly et al. (2010) with a maximum force of 3.3 N, **b** elastomeric tube in a woven fiber shell used in Polygerinos et al. (2015a), Zhang et al. (2018), Shiota et al. (2019) [maximum force: 8 N (Polygerinos et al. 2015a, b), 2.10 N (Zhang et al. 2018), 36.1 cNm (Shiota et al. 2019)], **c** elastomeric tube containing several channel cells used in Polygerinos et al. (2013), Zhao et al. (2015) [1.21 N (Polygerinos et al. 2013), 27.4 N (Zhao et al. 2015) using rotational casting system, 70.4 N (Yap et al. 2016a) with 3D printed Ninjaflex, 44.9 N (Ang and Yeow 2017) with 3D printed Ninjaflex], and **d** elastomeric tube with varied wall thickness (Yap et al. 2015a, b, c, 2016b, 2017) [maximum force: 3.59 N (Yap et al. 2015a, b, c), 13.6 N (Yap et al. 2016b), 9.12N (Yap et al. 2017)]

Using pneumatic or hydraulic actuation, hardware can be positioned remotely allowing the wearable device to be compact and simple-structured (Polygerinos et al. 2015a; Yap et al. 2015a). This feature also enables the development of Magnetic Resonance Imaging (MRI) compatible devices by keeping all electronics away from the operation site in surgical applications, e.g. applications in Functional Magnetic Resonance Imaging (fMRI) (Yap et al. 2015b); MR-compatible pneumatic and hydraulic soft hand exoskeletons can be integrated to fMRI to help study of the brain motor performance during rehabilitation.

Most wearable hand robots with soft materials are handmade. Several tedious steps such as making molds, material weighing and mixing fluidic elastomer components, degassing to reduce air bubbles and multi-stage casting processes are required to make a soft actuator (depending on the design complexity). Making soft actuators with complex inner geometry often requires careful, multi-part molds design. However, several innovative fabrication methods are proposed by researchers in this area implying that making 3D printable soft pneumatic actuators for wearable hand robots with soft materials is becoming less complicated; in 2016, a novel technique for 3D printing soft pneumatic actuators was proposed, allowing the fabrication of soft robots with complex architectures. This technique has been used in wearable robots for finger and wrist rehabilitation (Yap et al. 2016a). As shown in Fig. 2.2, 3D printable soft actuators can provide larger output force than other silicone rubber-based soft actuators made through casting processes (Yap et al. 2016a; Ang and Yeow 2017).

Wearable hand robots with soft materials suffer from several key drawbacks. The pneumatic and hydraulic actuation systems need devices such as fluid pump or reservoir that increase the weight and size of the whole system. Moreover, the hysteresis caused by the use of hyperplastic materials adds complexity to the design of the controller (Yap et al. 2015a). To improve wearable soft hand robots, new sensing tools such as pose and tactile sensors should be integrated into the soft body to improve the control accuracy as well as the human–robot interaction safety (Polygerinos et al. 2015a). Although providing bidirectional support, including both finger flexion and extension, is crucial for hand rehabilitation devices, as stroke patients tend to suffer from finger flexor tension (Thibaut et al. 2013; Iqbal et al. 2014), many current soft hand robots such as devices in Polygerinos et al. (2015a), Yap et al. (2015a) only provide finger flexion assistance. To support both the flexion and extension motions of fingers extra air chambers should be integrated (Yap et al. 2016a), increasing the hardware and control complexities. Therefore, clearly, there is a trade-off between the supported DOF and the system complexity. Whilst the abduction–adduction motion of fingers is essential for grasping, in most of the wearable hand robots based on soft materials, the thumb abduction–adduction is not fully supported. To rectify this, an active abduction–adduction DOF should be added for thumb actuation. Such a thumb actuator proposed by Kadowaki et al. (2011) comprises a spiral rubber muscle mechanism whereas Polygerinos et al. (2015a) used a similar bend-twist soft actuator for thumb actuation. Up to now, there is still a technological gap on devices that can provide assistance in abduction–adduction motion for other fingers. Therefore, this problem needs more research attention.

Tendon-Driven Mechanisms and Other Mechanisms

As shown in Fig. 2.3a, the human finger works via muscles, tendons, and annular ligaments (often referred as pulleys) acting on the hand skeleton (In et al. 2015). Wearable hand robots with tendon-driven mechanisms mimics the actuation of actual human fingers (Kim et al. 2022; Silva et al. 2023; Abdelhafiz et al. 2023). It has been observed that the design of tendon-driven wearable hand robots poses several different challenges. The challenges and proposed solutions by the research community are described as follows.

- Fabric gloves are often used as the base structure for tendon-driven wearable hand robots (Jeong et al. 2013). As the tendons apply shear forces to the attachment points an undesirable deformation of the fabric can be generated. As a solution to this problem, in In et al. (2015), a thimble-like strap mechanism was added to Exo-Glove for tendon attachment. Bagneschi et al. (2023) proposed a different tendon routing for the closing mechanism, folded laterally on both sides of the hand to enhance clenching forces when the exoskeleton is engaged to assist with grasping. This design improves glove stability and reduces tendon slippage or detachment from the palm during grasping tasks.
- Hand robots with tendon-driven mechanisms apply undesirable squeezing forces to user's hand causing discomfort. Ochoa et al. (2011) and Triandafilou et al.

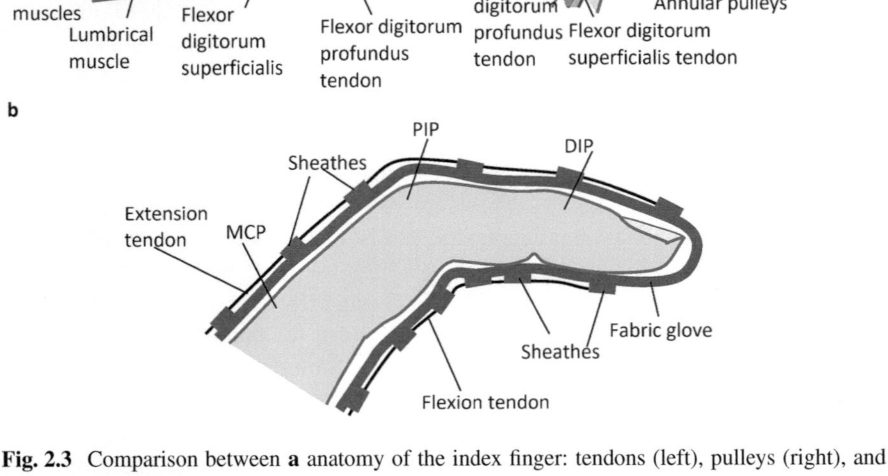

Fig. 2.3 Comparison between **a** anatomy of the index finger: tendons (left), pulleys (right), and **b** a commonly used tendon-driven mechanism of hand robot

(2014) reported on the development of J-glove and X-glove that integrate an array of plastic cable guides to the back of the glove which reduces the squeezing force applied to the back of the hand. Similarly, Popov et al. (2017) added a rigid plate to the hand robot to reduce the impact of the soft corset of the glove on cable squeezing force applied to the user's palm.
- The movement of all three joints in a finger should be coordinated to reflect natural flexion. However, through the commonly used design approach, described in Fig. 2.3b, the DIP joint of the finger initiates bending, followed by the PIP joint. The PIP joint remains extended until the DIP joint reaches its full range of motion, and likewise, the MCP joint begins to flex only after the PIP joint has reached its limit. Yang et al. (2016) proposed a tendon arrangement plan to achieve a more natural bending sequence for the finger joints. In this approach, a pair of staggered tendons (DPflex and PMflex) as well as an auxiliary tendon arrangement were added to maintain the coordinated movement of the DIP/PIP and PIP/MCP joints during finger extension and flexion, simulating the tendon system's function in the human finger shown in Fig. 2.3a.
- The use of the fabric glove in wearable hand robots faces limitations in multi-user applications because of the difficulty of sanitizing the fabric glove between uses. To overcome the sanitization problem in Exo-Glove Poly wearable hand robots, soft polymer materials were used instead of fabrics (Kang et al. 2016).
- In tendon-driven mechanisms, transmitting bi-directional movements is complex, since the wire only transmits the force uni-directionally. To enable bidirectional movement transmission, researchers developed a tendon-driven hand exoskeleton that functions like a tendon during extension, and as a compressed element that returns the wires to their original position (Borboni et al. 2016).
- The abduction–adduction motion of the fingers has not yet been supported for tendon-driven mechanisms.

Other Mechanisms

A number of hand robots using other mechanisms were also proposed. Arata et al. (2013) proposed a hand exoskeleton featuring a mechanism with three layers of sliding springs developed to support stroke patients experiencing hand muscle weakness while performing opening and closing actions. Nycz et al. (2016) and Butzer et al. (2021) extended this design to a remotely actuated one and used a Bowden cable to reduce the weight of the exoskeleton. Some researchers such as Jiang et al. (2018) and Stilli et al. (2018) attempted to combine wearable hand robots with soft materials and tendon-driven mechanisms to provide more motion patterns. Chen et al. (2022) proposed a hybrid actuation system that integrates tendon-driven actuation with a flexible linkage to achieve complex thumb movements, such as circumduction, utilizing only two actuators. Brogi et al. (2024) combined a linkage-based rigid architecture and a soft architecture with two flat springs to form a hybrid architecture for finger exoskeletons. Electro-Active Polymer (EAP) materials such as Ionic

Polymer Metal Composites (IPMCs) (Sareh et al. 2013) and Dielectric Elastomers (DE) can also be used to develop soft actuators. However, practical applications of EAPs are limited due to typically insufficient amount of force generated by these materials (Sareh et al. 2013) and, in some cases, the high driving voltage (usually >1 kV for DEs).

2.4 Sensing and Control of Soft Wearable Hand Robots

Movement Monitoring and Force Sensing

Movement monitoring and force sensing are required for precise control of hand exoskeletons, particularly for wearable hand robots based on soft materials. Motion capture (Mo-cap) systems, like VICON (Vicon Motion Systems, Ltd, Oxford, UK), which are based on high-speed cameras, are popular solutions for evaluating wearable hand robots. However, these systems are relatively expensive, often ineffective due to the optical occlusion and are mainly applicable to structured laboratory environments. Moreover, Mo-cap systems often require markers to be attached to the human body and involve time-consuming video motion analysis processes (Baker 2006). Electromagnetic tracking systems, such as the NDI Aurora (Northern Digital Inc., Canada) used in AirExGlove (Stilli et al. 2018) and TrakSTAR (Ascension Tech. Corp., Milton, VT, USA) used in the soft robotic glove described in Polygerinos et al. (2015a), can detect the positions and orientations of a limited number of magnetic tracking coils embedded within or attached to the hand robot. Nevertheless, these devices are also expensive, require construction of wearable hand robots from non-magnetic elements, and have limitations concerning the mobility of the magnetic field generation system (Sareh et al. 2015a). Data gloves are also another class of relevant technologies for motion sensing in fingers often based on flex sensors. However, data gloves can also be expensive, and force exerted by the tendon-driven and soft hand exoskeleton actuators on the data glove may affect data readings. Unlike the above solutions, soft stretch sensors can be integrated into the wearable robots and are typically lower cost. Off-the-shelf examples include conductive rubber-based stretch sensors (Images Scientific Instruments Inc, USA), which utilize simple resistive circuits to measure elongation. However, conductive rubber suffers from significant relaxation times and hysteresis effects. Another type of stretch sensor is based on dielectric elastomer technology, offered by companies such as StretchSense Ltd (New Zealand) and Danfoss PolyPower A/S (Denmark). Although separation of different sensing modes, such as pressure and stretch, is complex (Gisby et al. 2014), these sensors can accurately measure the stretch length through a near-linear voltage–length relationship. Sareh et al. (2015a, b), Sareh and Noh (2018) developed a stretch sensor using optical fibers that can measure the stretch length based on the principle that bending an optical fiber modulates the intensity of light transmitted through it. In 2022, Deng et al. (2022) proposed a Sen-Glove, integrated with fourteen soft strain sensors, with each sensor aligned to one of the fourteen joints in the five fingers. These strain sensors detect joint movements when the user passively or actively bends their fingers, enabling a gesture classification accuracy of 98.6% for eleven different hand gestures. A drawback with most examples of stretch sensors is the limited lifetime. The alignment difference between the hand joint and the sensor is another issue to overcome (Deng et al. 2022).

Flexible force sensors, such as the TakkStrip (Takktile LLC, USA) employed in Polygerinos et al. (2015b) as well as the Flexiforce (Tekscan Inc, USA) used in Yap et al. (2015a), are often attached ed to the back side of the finger or to the fingertips to acquire the contact interaction forces to be used for the evaluation of wearable hand robots. Apart from the human–robot interactive forces, human–environment interactive forces, such as fingertip force applied to grasped objects, or forces applied to the palm during grasping exercises, can be measured to provide better grasping assistance. For example, SEM glove measured the fingertip forces using several force-sensing resistors and the force applied to the palm using a series of integrated capacitive sensors (Nilsson et al. 2012).

Present systems for movement monitoring and force sensing rely predominantly on off-the-shelf sensors and actuator components that are not preserving the softness or flexibility of soft wearable hand robots. This highlights the need for further research into advanced robotic subsystems lightweight and compact enough, with appropriate geometries, to be seamlessly integrated into wearable devices.

Motion Planning in Soft Wearable Hand Robots

The motion patterns and strategies of fingers should be investigated and incorporated to the control of hand exoskeletons to achieve better conformity to the motion patterns of human fingers (Vaz et al. 2017). To achieve this goal, cubic polynomial interpolation and 3–4–5 polynomial interpolation methods are often used in the motion planning of hand robots with rigid structures. In Biggar and Yao (2016), the difference of percentage workload of the finger joints between soft wearable robot-driven hand motions and natural hand motions was noticed. There have been a number of efforts to achieve natural patterns of finger motions in soft wearable hand robots predominantly focused on the structural design aspects. For example, Yang et al. (2016) a new design for the tendon arrangement to achieve a more natural flexion sequence in human finger joints. Although, a substantial level of progress on the development of natural motion patterns is evident, the motion patterns and strategies used by the healthy people in ADLs, parameters such as the velocity and acceleration, are not fully understood and incorporated into the motion planning system of existing soft wearable hand robots yet. New research and development on identification, precise definition and generation of healthy reference trajectories and applying them to the design of soft wearable hand robots is desired with minimum increase in the complexity of the overall system. Ideally, the reference trajectories should be customized for users with different physical characteristics.

Control Algorithms of Soft Wearable Hand Robots

On one hand, compared to rigid exoskeletons, the flexibility of soft wearable hand robots introduces greater system nonlinearity, raising barriers to overcome in accurate position and motion control (Kang et al. 2016). On the other hand, to some extent, wearable hand robots do not require sophisticated protection or stability control algorithms as used in rigid exoskeletons thanks to the shock-absorbing characteristics of the materials employed (Lee et al. 2017). Therefore, open-loop control schemes, in which the necessary inputs are pre-determined and applied to the robot without monitoring its actual state, are still used in some soft wearable hand robots (Borboni et al. 2016; Popov et al. 2017; Kang et al. 2016). This type of control does not monitor when the actuator attains the target state, if it does so at all. Trial-and-error methods or a mathematical model of the actuator is required for open-loop control schemes (Polygerinos et al. 2017). For example, a Denavit–Hartenberg method was used in Popov et al. (2017).

However, to achieve a more precise control, the development of closed-loop control schemes that allow real-time correction of system dynamic response are needed. The closed-loop approach enables following a desired behavior based on a feedback loop using sensing signals. A simple "bang-bang controller", which keeps increasing the input until a desired flexion angle, position, or interactive force is exceeded and decreases the input otherwise, was used in Nycz et al. (2016). The majority of control algorithms used in soft wearable hand robots are classical control systems that use the Laplace transform as the main modelling tool to address the behavior of dynamic systems with inputs and adjust their behavior through the use of a feedback mechanism. The use of force or bending angle-based feedback control systems employing proportional-integral (PI), proportional-derivative (PD), or proportional-integral-derivative (PID) control algorithms is very common for wearable hand robots constructed with soft materials (Wang et al. 2017b; Haghshenas-Jaryani et al. 2016a, b, 2017). In some cases, the controlled variables such as the force or bending angles are converted to air or hydraulic pressure, and then air (hydraulic) pressure-based feedback control is performed (Polygerinos et al. 2013, 2015a; Wang et al. 2017a; Ang and Yeow 2017; Yap et al. 2016b, 2017; Maeder-York et al. 2014; Cappello et al. 2018b). The force or position-based feedback control using the PID control algorithm is commonly applied to a wide range of tendon-driven soft wearable hand robots (Arata et al. 2013; Nilsson et al. 2012; Park et al. 2016, 2018a, b).

In grasping assistance applications of tendon-driven wearable hand robots, impedance control is widely used to prevent sudden changes in the contact force applied and to ensure safe grasping (Jeong et al. 2013). Isotonic, isokinetic, and impedance control algorithms are commonly used in tendon-driven wearable hand robots for rehabilitation applications such as Exo-Glove, a soft exoskeleton designed to assist and enhance motor function in individuals with hand impairments (Jeong et al. 2013). Fuzzy control is also used in soft wearable hand robots (Al-fahaam et al. 2018a; Setiawan et al. 2021); different from other control algorithms, which operates using discrete values of either 0 or 1, fuzzy control processes the input signal in the form of logical variables whose continuous values are between 0 and 1. As people often use imprecise, non-numerical information to make decisions, the fuzzy control method suggests using fuzzy logic and models to represent and process imprecise information. The soft wearable hand robots are challenging to model due to the nonlinear properties of soft materials. Therefore, the fuzzy control can be used as an advanced control method to solve the nonlinear control problems associated with them (Nuchkrua and Leephakpreeda 2013; Židek et al. 2012) and to make the operation process more friendly to users. In addition, several soft wearable hand robots have been developed based on hybrid control strategies (Al-fahaam et al. 2018a; b) providing the user with additional reference information to enable more accurate and reliable motion control.

Motion Intention Sensing and Intuitive Control of Soft Wearable Hand Robots

User-friendly interfaces and intuitive control systems are critical for all applications of soft wearable hand robots, particularly in assistive and rehabilitation contexts. Accurate detection of a user's motion intention is vital for effective control, enabling the robot to seamlessly support or augment the user's movements (Heo et al. 2012). Research indicates that integrating intention with sensorimotor feedback during movement execution yields superior rehabilitation outcomes compared to passive movements or isolated stimulation (Mrachacz-Kersting et al. 2012; Takeuchi and Izumi 2013). This approach allows peripheral stimulation controlled by brain-computer interfaces to temporarily bypass impaired motor pathways, benefiting stroke patients with compromised movement execution.

Techniques that identify and translate motion intentions, muscular activities, and movement patterns into robotic actions facilitate intuitive control of wearable hand robots. Various kinematic and dynamic parameters—such as contact force, velocity, torque, joint angles, position, muscle hardness, photoplethysmography (PPG) at the fingernail (measuring changes in blood volume within the tissue's microvascular network), and finger pad deformation—can be employed to sense motion intention (Heo et al. 2012). For example, wrist motion has been used to trigger hand exoskeleton activation (In et al. 2015), while initial movements can be monitored to estimate grasping patterns (Toya et al. 2011). Bending angle sensors and pressure sensors provide non-invasive methods to detect user intent, but these techniques are unsuitable for patients with complete hand paralysis.

Electromyographic (EMG) signals have proven effective in detecting motor intent for use in tendon-driven and soft hand exoskeletons (Arata et al. 2013; Nycz et al. 2016; Delph et al. 2013). EMG-based methods reliably differentiate specific hand motions but require residual muscle activity, limiting their application for patients with complete paralysis. Additionally, in rehabilitation, high-level central nervous system damage may result in weakened EMG signals. Continuous EMG control also risks reinforcing pathological movement patterns rather than promoting the recovery of normal motion (Krebs et al. 2003).

Electroencephalography (EEG) provides an alternative for detecting motion intent, particularly in patients with complete paralysis, as intent signals are captured at the onset of motor pathway activity. EEG is non-invasive, portable, and relatively user-friendly compared to other neuroimaging methods (Nicolas-Alonso and Gomez-Gil 2012). For example, motor imagery-based EEG signals have been used to trigger finger extension assistance (McConnell et al. 2017). However, the low spatial resolution of EEG signals complicates the control of individual finger movements. Attenuation during signal transmission further hinders precise classification for movement control. To address these challenges, multimodal approaches combining EEG, EMG, and electrooculography (EOG) have been proposed, enabling more accurate control of soft robotic hands (Zhang et al. 2019).

Other emerging methods for motion intention sensing include force myography, which uses sensor bands with force-sensing resistors (FSRs) to monitor muscle contractions and relaxations, assessing hand motion states and muscle activity (Islam and Bai 2020). Voice commands are also being explored as intuitive control methods for soft wearable hand robots, offering a hands-free approach to device operation (Tran et al. 2020, 2022).

Despite these advances, significant challenges remain. EEG systems, for instance, are often costly and require time-consuming setup procedures, such as wearing EEG caps and applying conductive gel. For example, widely used device for acquiring EEG signals, the g.tec instrument from g.tec medical engineering GmbH (Schiedlberg, Austria), has a price tag exceeding US$10,000. The trade-offs among cost, user convenience, and signal stability need further exploration to improve practicality and accessibility. Future research should focus on optimizing these systems for affordability, ease of use, and reliable operation to enhance the overall effectiveness of soft wearable hand robots.

2.5 A 3D-Printed Soft Robotic Glove Capable of Assisting Finger Abduction

Existing hand rehabilitation devices predominantly focus on assisting finger flexion motions, often overlooking finger abduction. This limitation compromises the ability to support complex movements crucial for ADLs. Finger abduction, when combined with flexion, enables a broader range of functional hand movements. Current devices also often fail to control individual finger joints, which reduces their effectiveness in replicating natural, precise hand motions (Tong et al. 2010; Ueki et al. 2012). Pneumatic systems, in particular, frequently lack the capacity to separately control joint motions, further constraining their utility (Polygerinos et al. 2015a; Yap et al. 2015a).

Traditional fabrication methods for soft devices primarily rely on casting and molding, which can be complex processes. Mold design requires specialized expertise, and molds often need to be revised due to structural changes. Fortunately, 3D printing technology offers a new and more efficient fabrication approach. It enables the direct creation of intricate 3D models from digital designs, significantly reducing the time and effort involved in production (Aubin et al. 2014).

To address these challenges, we developed a 3D-printed soft robotic glove incorporating actuators for both finger flexion and abduction. This design not only provides targeted assistance for abduction motions but also ensures independent joint control for complex, realistic hand movements. The two soft glove designs discussed in this section were originally introduced in our prior conference papers (Li et al. 2019, 2020). In this chapter, we provide a side-by-side comparison and present reanalyzed data to highlight their relative performance under unified evaluation criteria.

Design and Fabrication

The normal maximum ROMs of human finger joints for thumb MCP, thumb IP, MCP, DIP, and PIP are 60°, 80°, 90°, 100°, and 80°, respectively. The actuators were designed for continuous passive motion (CPM) rehabilitation, a method shown to benefit patients with nerve damage (Hu et al. 2009). The glove supports flexion and abduction motions within a safe range, 2/3 of the normal ROMs of the joints (40°, 53°, 60°, 66°, and 53° for thumb MCP, thumb IP, MCP, DIP, and PIP, respectively), as advised by therapists from Xijing Hospital. The actuators' dimensions (maximum width and height: 20 mm) were minimized to avoid interference with finger movements. To ensure adequate performance, the actuators were required to generate forces exceeding 7.3 N and maintain a total device weight below 0.5 kg (Polygerinos et al. 2015a; Aubin et al. 2014).

The flexion actuators were tailored to accommodate the thumb's IP and MCP joints, as well as the MCP, PIP, and DIP joints of the other fingers. Abduction actuators were designed for motion between adjacent fingers, with each actuator independently controlled to facilitate combined flexion and abduction movements.

The glove integrates flexion actuators placed on the dorsal side of the fingers and abduction actuators positioned between adjacent fingers. Flexion actuators feature rigid components over knuckles to enhance bending efficiency and soft components over joints for flexibility. Abduction actuators employ asymmetrical cavity designs, enabling targeted deformation under pressurization.

When actuated, the pressurized cavities of the soft actuators induce deformation, allowing precise assistance for flexion and abduction motions. Negative pressure facilitates the actuators' return to their original state. Two types of flexion actuators with a square (type I) (Li et al. 2019) and a semicircular cross-section shape (type II) (Li et al. 2020) were designed. These components were modeled in SolidWorks, with 3D models depicted in Fig. 2.4.

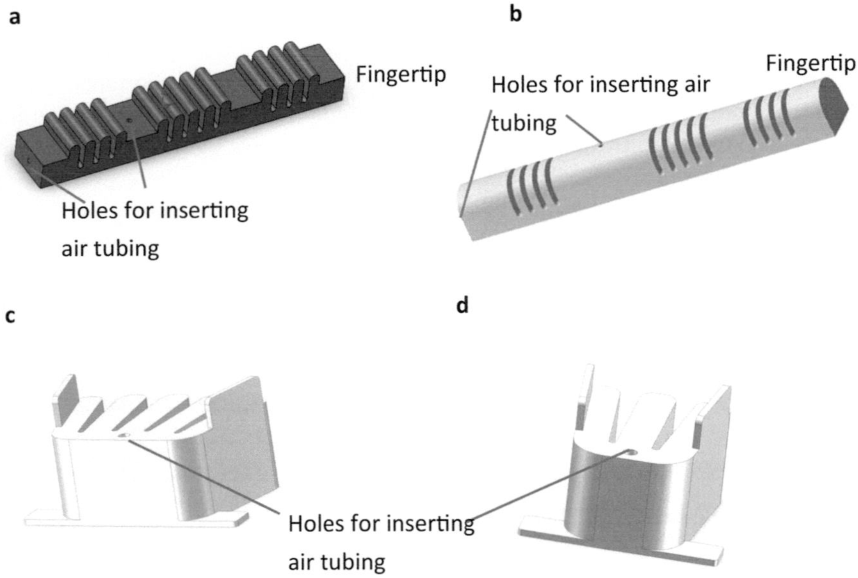

Fig. 2.4 The 3D models of actuators: **a** index flexion actuator of type I, **b** index flexion actuator of type II, **c** abduction actuator for thumb/index fingers, and **d** abduction actuator for other adjacent fingers

As presented in our previous work (Li et al. 2019, 2020), the actuators were fabricated using NinjaFlex 85A TPU material on a LulzBot TAZ 6 desktop 3D printer (Fargo Additive Manufacturing Equipment 3D, LLC, Fargo, ND, USA) with customized parameters. Key differences between Type I and Type II actuators include:

- Type I: Layer height of 0.1 mm, initial layer height of 0.5 mm, shell thickness of 1.0 mm, and 100% infill density.
- Type II: Layer height of 0.4 mm, initial layer height of 0.4 mm, shell thickness of 0.5 mm, and 70% infill density.

Both types shared an extrusion width of 0.5 mm and a nozzle temperature of 230 °C. The infill overlap varied significantly, though the exact value for Type I was not specified. Assembly involved attaching rigid flexion actuator components using Velcro and securing air tubes to the actuators with silicone sealant (RTV108). The final gloves weighed 0.172 kg for Type I and 0.144 kg for Type II, both well below the target weight of 0.5 kg.

Experimental Evaluation

Flexion Motion

As shown in our previous research (Li et al. 2019), the ROM for the Type I glove was evaluated using a Vicon motion capture system. A healthy subject wore the glove while minimizing voluntary hand effort, and infrared markers attached to the glove tracked finger flexion. At an actuator pressure of 0.30 MPa, multi-joint flexion was achieved, and the resulting maximum joint angles are reported in Table 2.1. In contrast, the ROM of the Type II actuators was assessed in vitro in our prior study (Li et al. 2020). Each actuator was secured with a jaw clamp during testing, and deformation was recorded by a camera as pressure was incrementally increased from 0 to 0.30 MPa. Joint angles were extracted through image analysis, and the results are also summarized in Table 2.1. The comparison revealed that the maximum flexion angles achieved by the type I actuators, when worn by a subject, were smaller than those of the type II actuators evaluated separately. This discrepancy is likely due to the constraints imposed by wearing the glove, including anatomical limitations and interaction with the human hand.

As detailed in our previous work (Li et al. 2019, 2020), a 40 mm-diameter polylactic acid (PLA) cylinder was used to evaluate the grasping force of the actuators. For the Type I actuator, pressurized to 0.30 MPa and secured with a jaw clamp, a hoisting mechanism gradually lifted the cylinder until grip failure occurred. The exerted force was recorded using a BBTGTJL-1 force sensor. Given the identical design of the index and ring finger actuators, their performance was assessed together. Each test was repeated three times for consistency. The maximum individual actuator forces were 8.9 N (thumb to ring finger) and 9.2 N (little finger) (Li et al. 2019), yielding a total maximum force of 44.8 N—exceeding the 7.3 N threshold required for most daily activities (Polygerinos et al. 2015a).

The same setup was used to test the Type II actuator. The individual finger forces (from little to thumb) were 9.1, 6.6, 5.9, 7.6, and 7.7 N, respectively (Li et al. 2020). While some actuators fell below the 7.3 N per-finger threshold, the combined

Table 2.1 Maximum flexion angles of flexion actuators across different fingers

Finger	MCP/°	PIP/°	DIP/°	IP/°
Thumb (type I/type II)	34.19/80.10	NA	NA	54.20/97.23
Index finger (type I/type II)	36.29/101.80	49.50/89.20	61.14/92.47	NA
Middle finger (type I/type II)	41.91/101.13	78.07/90.40	58.43/72.70	NA
Ring finger (type I/type II)	50.98/100.70	56.96/98.87	51.39/80.30	NA
Pinky finger (type I/type II)	41.07/93.7	82.40/86.00	78.56/83.57	NA

Data combined and reformatted from our previous works (Li et al. 2019, 2020).

maximum force reached 36.9 N, well above the 15 N requirement for functional grasping tasks (Polygerinos et al. 2015a).

Abduction Motion

Both glove types employed identical abduction actuators. As previously reported (Li et al. 2019), their performance was evaluated by measuring the maximum abduction angle as input pressure increased from 0.10 to 0.40 MPa, using an electronic protractor. When activated individually, the joint angles for the little/ring, ring/middle, middle/index, and index/thumb pairs (34.0°, 34.6°, 37.7°, and 69.4°) were greater than those achieved with all five actuators activated simultaneously (31.1°, 27.6°, 31.5°, and 51.3°). All values exceeded two-thirds of the normal range of motion (ROM)—50.0° for thumb/index and 25.0° for the others—demonstrating effective support for both isolated and concurrent finger abduction, with strong potential for rehabilitation applications.

Abduction forces were also measured over the same pressure range using a Nano17 force sensor (SI-12-0.12, ATI, USA), with actuators secured in a custom 3D-printed fixture. At 0.40 MPa, the maximum output force was 15.00 N for the thumb and index fingers and 10.70 N for the others (Li et al. 2019). All actuators delivered forces exceeding 10 N, confirming their capability to provide sufficient mechanical assistance for functional rehabilitation tasks.

Post-Wearing Motion Assessment of the Gloves

To evaluate the practical functionality of the gloves, their ability to perform complex rehabilitation movements was tested using a data glove (Wise-Glove14, Xintianshijing Technology, China) as a control interface (see Fig. 2.5). The device demonstrated effective assistance by combining flexion and abduction motions, enabling activities of daily living (ADLs) with objects of varying shapes and stiffnesses.

The intrinsic delay characteristic of the rehabilitation training system might impact the user's comprehensive experience. To assess the system delay, a participant was asked to perform a forceful grasping motion seven consecutive times, with a 5-s rest period between each repetition to allow muscle relaxation. The entire experiment was recorded using an Android smartphone, and the time delay between each movement was analyzed frame by frame. A frame rate of 30 fps was used to record the video. The average delay for the type II glove was calculated as 0.8 ± 0.15 s. Given that rehabilitation training typically requires slow, controlled hand movements, this level of delay is within acceptable limits for effective training.

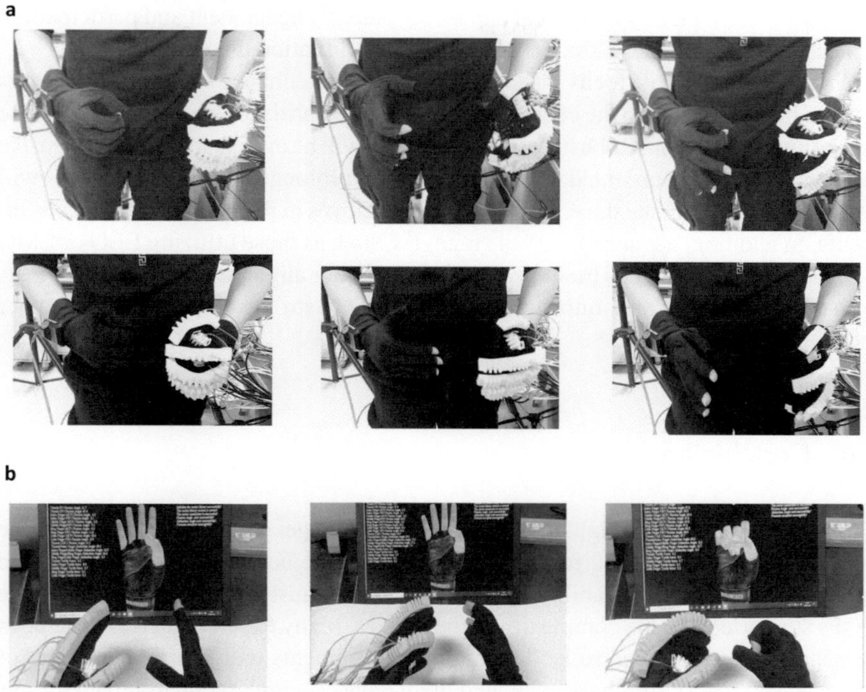

Fig. 2.5 Rehabilitation motion that could achieved using **a** type I glove and **b** type II glove

Discussion

Traditional manufacturing methods for flexible actuators, such as cast molding, involve complex processes that require the creation of molds, leading to longer production times and increased complexity. In contrast, the proposed gloves leverage 3D printing technology, which eliminates the need for mold formation. By directly printing the 3D model, this approach simplifies the manufacturing process, significantly improving efficiency and enabling greater customization.

The soft robotic gloves introduced in this study effectively provide assistance for both finger abduction and flexion, addressing limitations found in existing devices. Their lightweight design and use of 3D printing further enhance their practicality and adaptability. However, the current design supports only uni-directional flexion. Future iterations should incorporate bi-directional actuation, enabling both flexion and extension, which are essential for comprehensive hand rehabilitation (Iqbal et al. 2014).

The data glove-based collaborative treatment mode presents a promising approach for rehabilitation. For patients with hemiplegia, the ability to control the affected hand using the healthy hand facilitates rehabilitation training. Similarly, this method allows for bilateral training under the supervision of rehabilitation professionals, reducing the complexity of use and enhancing patient engagement and participation. This collaborative mode ultimately improves rehabilitation outcomes.

Future research will focus on several key areas to enhance the proposed gloves further. Improvements to the control system will be prioritized to ensure more precise and intuitive operation. Robustness and durability will be evaluated through extensive fatigue testing to ensure the device's reliability in prolonged use. Clinical trials will be conducted to evaluate the effectiveness of the gloves in real rehabilitation environments. In addition, advanced control strategies, such as those utilizing EEG or EMG signals, will be explored. These strategies aim to better align the device's movements with the user's intent, maximizing its effectiveness in stroke rehabilitation and other therapeutic applications.

2.6 Conclusion

The reviewed literature highlights significant challenges and advancements in the field of soft wearable hand robotics, underscoring the need for further research to enhance their practical usability. A critical balance must be achieved between the DOFs supported and the complexity of the system. Many existing devices have been demonstrated only in controlled laboratory environments with a limited number of subjects, and few studies have evaluated these devices with larger participant groups or over extended periods.

Moreover, the aesthetic design and ergonomics of soft wearable hand robots remain underexplored, despite their importance for user acceptance and long-term use. Addressing these gaps requires more comprehensive studies on human motion patterns and control strategies, as well as the development of advanced motion tracking and force sensing systems tailored to the characteristics of soft wearable devices. Thorough evaluation studies involving diverse user groups and long-term trials are essential to establish the efficacy and reliability of these robots.

Future research should also focus on innovative materials and fabrication technologies to improve electromechanical integration and optimize user comfort. By addressing these challenges, the next generation of soft wearable hand robots can provide more effective, practical, and user-friendly solutions for rehabilitation and assistive applications.

References

Abdelhafiz MH, Andreasen-Struijk LNS, Dosen S, Spaich EG (2023) Biomimetic tendon-based mechanism for finger flexion and extension in a soft hand exoskeleton: design and experimental assessment. Sensors 23:2272. https://doi.org/10.3390/s23042272

Al-fahaam H, Davis S, Theo SN (2018a) Novel soft bending actuator-based power augmentation hand exoskeleton controlled by human intention. Intell Serv Robot 11:247–268. https://doi.org/10.1007/s11370-018-0250-4

Al-Fahaam H, Davis S, Nefti-Meziani S (2018b) The design and mathematical modelling of novel extensor bending pneumatic artificial muscles (EBPAMs) for soft exoskeletons. Rob Auton Syst 99:63–74. https://doi.org/10.1016/j.robot.2017.10.010

Ang BWK, Yeow C-H (2017) Print-it-yourself (PIY) glove: a fully 3D printed soft robotic hand rehabilitative and assistive exoskeleton for stroke patients. In: Proceedings of the 2017 IEEE/RSJ international conference on intelligent robots and systems (IROS). IEEE, pp 1219–1223

Arata J, Ohmoto K, Gassert R et al (2013) A new hand exoskeleton device for rehabilitation using a three-layered sliding spring mechanism. Proc IEEE Int Conf Robot Autom 14:3902–3907. https://doi.org/10.1109/ICRA.2013.6631126

Aubin P, Petersen K, Sallum H et al (2014) A pediatric robotic thumb exoskeleton for at-home rehabilitation. Int J Intell Comput Cybern 7:233–252. https://doi.org/10.1108/IJICC-10-2013-0043

Bagneschi T, Chiaradia D, Righi G et al (2023) A soft hand exoskeleton with a novel tendon layout to improve stable wearing in grasping assistance. IEEE Trans Hapt 16:311–321. https://doi.org/10.1109/TOH.2023.3273908

Baker R (2006) Gait analysis methods in rehabilitation. J Neuroeng Rehabil 3:4. https://doi.org/10.1186/1743-0003-3-4

Beer RF, Ellis MD, Holubar BG, Dewald JPA (2007) Impact of gravity loading on post-stroke reaching and its relationship to weakness. Muscle Nerve 36:242–250. https://doi.org/10.1002/mus.20817

Bianchi M, Cempini M, Conti R et al (2018) Design of a series elastic transmission for hand exoskeletons. Mechatronics 51:8–18. https://doi.org/10.1016/j.mechatronics.2018.02.010

Biggar S, Yao W (2016) Design and evaluation of a soft and wearable robotic glove for hand rehabilitation. IEEE Trans Neural Syst Rehabil Eng 24:1071–1080. https://doi.org/10.1109/TNSRE.2016.2521544

Borboni A, Mor M, Faglia R (2016) Gloreha—hand robotic rehabilitation: design, mechanical model, and experiments. J Dyn Syst Meas Control 138:111003. https://doi.org/10.1115/1.4033831

Bouzit M, Burdea G, Popescu G, Boian R (2002) The Rutgers master II—new design force-feedback glove. IEEE/ASME Trans Mechatr 7:256–263. https://doi.org/10.1109/TMECH.2002.1011262

Brogi C, Secciani N, Bartalucci L et al (2024) An original hybrid-architecture finger mechanism for wearable hand exoskeletons. Mechatronics 98:103117. https://doi.org/10.1016/j.mechatronics.2023.103117

Bützer T, Lambercy O, Arata J, Gassert R (2021) Fully wearable actuated soft exoskeleton for grasping assistance in everyday activities. Soft Robot 8:128–143. https://doi.org/10.1089/soro.2019.0135

Cappello L, Galloway KC, Sanan S et al (2018a) Exploiting textile mechanical anisotropy for fabric-based pneumatic actuators. Soft Robot 5:662–674. https://doi.org/10.1089/soro.2017.0076

Cappello L, Meyer JT, Galloway KC et al (2018b) Assisting hand function after spinal cord injury with a fabric-based soft robotic glove. J Neuroeng Rehabil 15:1–10. https://doi.org/10.1186/s12984-018-0391-x

Chen W, Li G, Li N et al (2022) Soft exoskeleton with fully actuated thumb movements for grasping assistance. IEEE Trans Robot 38:2194–2207. https://doi.org/10.1109/TRO.2022.3148909

Chiri A, Vitiello N, Giovacchini F et al (2012) Mechatronic design and characterization of the index finger module of a hand exoskeleton for post-stroke rehabilitation. IEEE/ASME Trans Mechatr 17:884–894. https://doi.org/10.1109/TMECH.2011.2144614

Chu CY, Patterson RM (2018) Soft robotic devices for hand rehabilitation and assistance: a narrative review. J Neuroeng Rehabil 15:1–14. https://doi.org/10.1186/s12984-018-0350-6

Connelly L, Jia Y, Toro ML et al (2010) A pneumatic glove and immersive virtual reality environment for hand rehabilitative training after stroke. IEEE Trans Neural Syst Rehabil Eng 18:551–559. https://doi.org/10.1109/TNSRE.2010.2047588

Cui L, Phan A, Allison G (2015) Design and fabrication of a three dimensional printable non-assembly articulated hand exoskeleton for rehabilitation. In: International conference of the IEEE engineering in medicine and biology society, pp 4627–4630

Dai JS, Delun W, Cui L (2009) Orientation and workspace analysis of the multifingered metamorphic hand—metahand. IEEE Trans Robot 25:942–947. https://doi.org/10.1109/TRO.2009.2017138

Delph MA, Fischer SA, Gauthier PW et al (2013) A soft robotic exomusculature glove with integrated sEMG sensing for hand rehabilitation. IEEE Int Confer Rehabil Robot 16:1–7

Deng L, Shen Y, Hong Y et al (2022) Sen-glove: a lightweight wearable glove for hand assistance with soft joint sensing. In: Proceedings of the 2022 international conference on robotics and automation (ICRA). IEEE, pp 5170–5175

Fang H, Xie Z, Liu H (2009) An exoskeleton master hand for controlling DLR/HIT hand. In: Proceedings of the 2009 IEEE/RSJ international conference on intelligent robots and systems, IROS 2009, pp 3703–3708

Gasser BW, Goldfarb M (2015) Design and performance characterization of a hand orthosis prototype to aid activities of daily living in a post-stroke population. In: Proceedings of the annual international conference of the IEEE engineering in medicine and biology society, EMBS. Institute of Electrical and Electronics Engineers Inc., pp 3877–3880

Gisby T, Anderson I, Limited S et al (2014) Stretch sensors for human body motion. Electroact Polym Actuat Dev. 9056:1–9. https://doi.org/10.1117/12.2046143

Go AS, Mozaffarian D, Roger VL et al (2014) Heart disease and stroke statistics—2014 update: a report from the American heart association. Circulation 129:e28–e292. https://doi.org/10.1161/01.cir.0000441139.02102.80

Haghshenas-Jaryani M, Carrigan W, Nothnagle C, Wijesundara MBJ (2016a) Sensorized soft robotic glove for continuous passive motion therapy. In: Proceedings of the IEEE RAS and EMBS international conference on biomedical robotics and biomechatronics. IEEE, pp 815–820

Haghshenas-Jaryani M, Carrigan W, Wijesundara MBJ et al (2016b) Kinematic study of a soft-and-rigid robotic digit for rehabilitation and assistive applications. In: ASME 2016 international design engineering technical conferences and computers and information in engineering conference, p V05BT07A065

Haghshenas-Jaryani M, Nothnagle C, Patterson RM, Bugnariu N, Wijesundara MBJ (2017) Soft robotic rehabilitation exoskeleton (REHAB glove) for hand therapy. In: ASME 2017 international design engineering technical conferences and computers and information in engineering conference, p V003T13A005

Heo P, Gu GM, Lee S et al (2012) Current hand exoskeleton technologies for rehabilitation and assistive engineering. Int J Precis Eng Manufact 13:807–824. https://doi.org/10.1007/s12541-012-0107-2

Hernandez-Barraza L, Fraiszudeen A, Yuan-Lee DL, Chen-Hua YR (2023) Development of a novel hybrid securing actuator for a self-securing soft robotic hand exoskeleton. Front Robot AI 10:1164819. https://doi.org/10.3389/frobt.2023.1164819

Ho NSK, Tong KY, Hu XL et al (2011) An EMG-driven exoskeleton hand robotic training device on chronic stroke subjects: task training system for stroke rehabilitation. In: Proceedings of the 2011 IEEE international conference on rehabilitation robotics. IEEE, pp 1–5

Hu XL, Tong KY, Song R et al (2009) A comparison between electromyography-driven robot and passive motion device on wrist rehabilitation for chronic stroke. Neurorehabil Neural Repair 23:837–846. https://doi.org/10.1177/1545968309338191

In H, Kang BK, Sin M, Cho K (2015) Exo-Glove: a soft wearable robot for the hand using soft tendon routing system. IEEE Robot Autom 22:97–105. https://doi.org/10.1109/MRA.2014.2362863

Iqbal J, Khan H, Tsagarakis NG, Caldwell DG (2014) A novel exoskeleton robotic system for hand rehabilitation: conceptualization to prototyping. Biocybern Biomed Eng 34:79–89. https://doi.org/10.1016/j.bbe.2014.01.003

Islam MRU, Bai S (2020) Effective multi-mode grasping assistance control of a soft hand exoskeleton using force myography. Front Robot AI 7:567491. https://doi.org/10.3389/frobt.2020.567491

Ito S, Kawasaki H, Ishigure Y et al (2011) A design of fine motion assist equipment for disabled hand in robotic rehabilitation system. J Franklin Inst 348:79–89. https://doi.org/10.1016/j.jfranklin.2009.02.009

Jeong U, In HK, Cho KJ (2013) Implementation of various control algorithms for hand rehabilitation exercise using wearable robotic hand. Intell Serv Robot 6:181–189. https://doi.org/10.1007/s11370-013-0135-5

Jiang Y, Chen D, Liu P et al (2018) Fishbone-inspired soft robotic glove for hand rehabilitation with multi-degrees-of-freedom. In: Proceedings of the 2018 IEEE international conference on soft robotics, RoboSoft 2018, pp 394–399

Jo I, Bae J (2017) Design and control of a wearable and force-controllable hand exoskeleton system. Mechatronics 41:90–101. https://doi.org/10.1016/j.mechatronics.2016.12.001

Kadowaki Y, Noritsugu T, Takaiwa M et al (2011) Development of soft power-assist glove and control based on human intent. J Robot Mechatr 23:281–291

Kamper DG, Fischer HC, Cruz EG, Rymer WZ (2006) Weakness is the primary contributor to finger impairment in chronic stroke. Arch Phys Med Rehabil 87:1262–1269. https://doi.org/10.1016/j.apmr.2006.05.013

Kang BB, Lee H, In H et al (2016) Development of a polymer-based tendon-driven wearable robotic hand. In: Proceedings—IEEE international conference on robotics and automation, pp 3750–3755

Kim DH, Lee Y, Park HS (2022) Bioinspired high-degrees of freedom soft robotic glove for restoring versatile and comfortable manipulation. Soft Robot 9:167. https://doi.org/10.1089/soro.2020.0167

Koyama T, Yamano I, Takemura K, Maeno T (2002) Multi-fingered exoskeleton haptic device using passive force feedback for dexterous teleoperation. In: Proceedings of the IEEE/RSJ international conference on intelligent robots and systems, pp 2905–2910

Krebs HI, Palazzolo JJ, Dipietro L et al (2003) Rehabilitation robotics: performance-based progressive robot-assisted therapy. Auton Robots 15:7–20

Lambercy O, Dovat L, Yun H et al (2011) Effects of a robot-assisted training of grasp and pronation/supination in chronic stroke: a pilot study. J Neuroeng Rehabil 8:63. https://doi.org/10.1186/1743-0003-8-63

Laschi C, Mazzolai B, Cianchetti M (2016) Soft robotics: technologies and systems pushing the boundaries of robot abilities. Sci Robot 1:1–12. https://doi.org/10.1126/scirobotics.aah3690

Lee C, Kim M, Kim YJ et al (2017) Soft robot review. Int J Control Autom Syst 15:1–13. https://doi.org/10.1007/s12555-016-0462-3

Li M, Ranzani T, Sareh S et al (2014a) Multi-fingered haptic palpation utilizing granular jamming stiffness feedback actuators. Smart Mater Struct 23:095007. https://doi.org/10.1088/0964-1726/23/9/095007

Li M, Luo S, Nanayakkara T et al (2014b) Multi-fingered haptic palpation using pneumatic feedback actuators. Sens Actuat A Phys 218:132–141. https://doi.org/10.1016/j.sna.2014.08.003

Li M, Zhuo Y, He B et al (2019) A 3D-printed soft hand exoskeleton with finger abduction assistance. In: Proceedings of the 2019 16th international conference on ubiquitous robots (UR). IEEE, pp 319–322

Li M, Wang T, Zhuo Y et al (2020) A soft robotic glove for hand rehabilitation training controlled by movements of the healthy hand. In: Proceedings of the 2020 17th international conference on ubiquitous robots, UR 2020

Maeder-York P, Clites T, Boggs E et al (2014) Biologically inspired soft robot for thumb rehabilitation. J Med Dev 8:020934. https://doi.org/10.1115/1.4027031

Maldonado-Mejía JC, Múnera M, Diaz CAR et al (2023) A fabric-based soft hand exoskeleton for assistance: the ExHand Exoskeleton. Front Neurorobot 17:1091827. https://doi.org/10.3389/fnbot.2023.1091827

Matheus K, Dollar AM (2010) Benchmarking grasping and manipulation: properties of the objects of daily living. In: IEEE/RSJ 2010 international conference on intelligent robots and systems, IROS 2010—conference proceedings, pp 5020–5027

McConnell AC, Vallejo M, Moioli RC et al (2017) SOPHIA: soft orthotic physiotherapy hand interactive aid. Front Mech Eng 3:1–13. https://doi.org/10.3389/fmech.2017.00003

Mrachacz-Kersting N, Kristensen SR, Niazi IK, Farina D (2012) Precise temporal association between cortical potentials evoked by motor imagination and afference induces cortical plasticity. J Physiol 590:1669–1682. https://doi.org/10.1113/jphysiol.2011.222851

Nassour J, Hamker FH, Cheng G (2020) High-performance perpendicularly-enfolded-textile actuators for soft wearable robots: design and realization. IEEE Trans Med Robot Bionics 2:309–319. https://doi.org/10.1109/TMRB.2020.3012131

Nicolas-Alonso LF, Gomez-Gil J (2012) Brain computer interfaces, a review. Sensors 12:1211–1279. https://doi.org/10.3390/s120201211

Nilsson M, Ingvast J, Wikander J, Von Holst H (2012) The soft extra muscle system for improving the grasping capability in neurological rehabilitation. In: Proceedings of the 2012 IEEE-EMBS conference on biomedical engineering and sciences, IECBES 2012. IEEE, pp 412–417

Nuchkrua T, Leephakpreeda T (2013) Fuzzy self-tuning PID control of hydrogen-driven pneumatic artificial muscle actuator. J Bionic Eng 10:329–340. https://doi.org/10.1016/S1672-6529(13)60228-0

Nycz CJ, Butzer T, Lambercy O et al (2016) Design and characterization of a lightweight and fully portable remote actuation system for use with a hand exoskeleton. IEEE Robot Autom Lett 1:976–983. https://doi.org/10.1109/LRA.2016.2528296

Ochoa JM, Kamper DG, Listenberger M, Lee SW (2011) Use of an electromyographically driven hand orthosis for training after stroke. IEEE Int Confer Rehabil Robot 16:5382. https://doi.org/10.1109/ICORR.2011.5975382

Park S, Bishop L, Post T et al (2016) On the feasibility of wearable exotendon networks for whole-hand movement patterns in stroke patients. In: Proceedings of the 2016 IEEE international conference on robotics and automation (ICRA). IEEE, pp 3729–3735

Park Y, Jo I, Lee J, Bae J (2018a) A dual-cable hand exoskeleton system for virtual reality. Mechatronics 49:177–186. https://doi.org/10.1016/j.mechatronics.2017.12.008

Park S, Weber L, Bishop L et al (2018b) Design and development of effective transmission mechanisms on a tendon driven hand orthosis for stroke patients. In: Proceedings of the 2018 IEEE international conference on robotics and automation (ICRA). IEEE, pp 2281–2287

Perry JC, Rosen J, Burns S (2007) Upper-limb powered exoskeleton design. IEEE/ASME Trans Mechatr 12:408–417. https://doi.org/10.1109/TMECH.2007.901934

Polygerinos P, Correll N, Morin SA et al (2017) Soft robotics: review of fluid-driven intrinsically soft devices; manufacturing, sensing, control, and applications in human–robot interaction. Adv Eng Mater 19:1700016. https://doi.org/10.1002/adem.201700016

Polygerinos P, Lyne S, Wang Z et al (2013) Towards a soft pneumatic glove for hand rehabilitation. In: IEEE international conference on intelligent robots and systems, pp 1512–1517

Polygerinos P, Wang Z, Galloway KC et al (2015a) Soft robotic glove for combined assistance and at-home rehabilitation. Rob Auton Syst 73:135–143. https://doi.org/10.1016/j.robot.2014.08.014

Polygerinos P, Wang Z, Galloway KC et al (2015b) Soft robotic glove for hand rehabilitation and task specific training. In: IEEE international conference on robotics and automation ICRA, pp 2913–2919

Popov D, Gaponov I, Ryu J-H (2017) Portable exoskeleton glove with soft structure for hand assistance in activities of daily living. IEEE/ASME Trans Mechatr 22:865–875. https://doi.org/10.1109/TMECH.2016.2641932

Prange GB, Jannink MJ, Groothuis-Oudshoorn CGM et al (2006) Systematic review of the effect of robot-aided therapy on recovery of the hemiparetic arm after stroke. J Rehabil Res Dev 43:171–184

Radder B, Prange-Lasonder GB, Kottink AIR et al (2020) The effect of a wearable soft-robotic glove on motor function and functional performance of older adults. Assist Technol 32:9–15. https://doi.org/10.1080/10400435.2018.1453888

Ramos O, Múnera M, Moazen M et al (2022) Assessment of soft actuators for hand exoskeletons: pleated textile actuators and fiber-reinforced silicone actuators. Front Bioeng Biotechnol 10:924888. https://doi.org/10.3389/fbioe.2022.924888

Reinkensmeyer DJ, Emken JL, Cramer SC (2004) Robotics, motor learning, and neurologic recovery. Annu Rev Biomed Eng 6:497–525. https://doi.org/10.1146/annurev.bioeng.6.040803.140223

Rus D, Tolley MT (2015) Design, fabrication and control of soft robots. Nature 521:467–475. https://doi.org/10.1038/nature14543

Ryu D, Moon K, Nam H et al (2008) Micro hydraulic system using slim artificial muscles for a wearable haptic glove. In: IEEE/RSJ international conference on intelligent robots and systems, pp 22–26

Sandoval-gonzalez O, Jacinto-villegas J, Herrera-aguilar I et al (2016) Design and development of a hand exoskeleton robot for active and passive rehabilitation. Int J Adv Robot Syst 13:66. https://doi.org/10.5772/62404

Sareh S, Rossiter J, Conn A et al (2013) Swimming like algae: biomimetic soft artificial cilia. J R Soc Interf 10:20120666. https://doi.org/10.1098/rsif.2012.0666

Sareh S, Noh Y (2018) Low profile stretch sensor for soft wearable robotics. In: Proceedings of the 2018 IEEE international conference on soft robotics (RoboSoft). IEEE, pp 479–484

Sareh S, Noh Y, Li M et al (2015a) Macrobend optical sensing for pose measurement in soft robot arms. Smart Mater Struct 24:125024. https://doi.org/10.1088/0964-1726/24/12/125024

Sareh S, Noh Y, Ranzani T et al (2015b) A 7.5 mm steiner chain fibre-optic system for multi-segment flex sensing. In: Proceedings of the 2015 IEEE/RSJ international conference on intelligent robots and systems (IROS). IEEE, pp 2336–2341

Setiawan JD, Ariyanto M, Nugroho S et al (2021) Fuzzy logic control for a soft exoskeleton glove using a motor-tendon actuator. Ingenieria e Investigacion 41:531

Shiota K, Kokubu S, Tarvainen TVJ et al (2019) Enhanced Kapandji test evaluation of a soft robotic thumb rehabilitation device by developing a fiber-reinforced elastomer-actuator based 5-digit assist system. Rob Auton Syst 111:20–30. https://doi.org/10.1016/j.robot.2018.09.007

Silva RC, BrunoG L, Ulhoa PHF et al (2023) Biomimetic design of a tendon-driven myoelectric soft hand exoskeleton for upper-limb rehabilitation. Biomimetics 8:317. https://doi.org/10.3390/biomimetics8030317

Smaby N, Johanson ME, Baker B et al (2004) Identification of key pinch forces required to complete functional tasks. J Rehabil Res Develop 41:215. https://doi.org/10.1682/JRRD.2004.02.0215

Stilli A, Cremoni A, Bianchi M et al (2018) AirExGlove: a novel pneumatic exoskeleton glove for adaptive hand rehabilitation in post-stroke patients. In: Proceedings of the 2018 IEEE international conference on soft robotics, RoboSoft 2018, pp 579–584

Suulker C, Skach S, Althoefer K (2022) Soft robotic fabric actuator with elastic bands for high force and bending performance in hand exoskeletons. IEEE Robot Autom Lett 7:10621–10627. https://doi.org/10.1109/LRA.2022.3194883

Takeuchi N, Izumi S-I (2013) Rehabilitation with Poststroke motor recovery: a review with a focus on neural plasticity. Stroke Res Treat 2013:128641. https://doi.org/10.1155/2013/128641

Thibaut A, Chatelle C, Ziegler E et al (2013) Spasticity after stroke: physiology, assessment and treatment. Brain Inj 27:1093–1105. https://doi.org/10.3109/02699052.2013.804202

Tong KY, Ho SK, Pang PMK et al (2010) An intention driven hand functions task training robotic system. In: Proceedings of the 2010 annual international conference of the IEEE engineering in medicine and biology society, EMBC'10, pp 3406–3409. https://doi.org/10.1109/IEMBS.2010.5627930

Toya K, Miyagawa T, Kubota Y (2011) Power-assist glove operated by predicting the grasping mode. J Syst des Dyn 5:94–108. https://doi.org/10.1299/jsdd.5.94

Tran P, Jeong S, Wolf SL, Desai JP (2020) Patient-specific, voice-controlled, robotic FLEXotendon glove-II system for spinal cord injury. IEEE Robot Autom Lett 5:898–905. https://doi.org/10.1109/LRA.2020.2965900

Tran P, Jeong S, Lyu F et al (2022) FLEXotendon glove-III: voice-controlled soft robotic hand exoskeleton with novel fabrication method and admittance grasping control. IEEE/ASME Trans Mechatr 27:3920–3931. https://doi.org/10.1109/TMECH.2022.3148032

Triandafilou KM, Ochoa JM, Kamper DG (2014) Effect of static versus cyclical stretch on hand motor control in subacute stroke. Int J Neurorehabil 1:1–5. https://doi.org/10.4172/ijn.1000124

Ueki S, Kawasaki H, Ito S et al (2012) Development of a hand-assist robot with multi-degrees-of-freedom for rehabilitation therapy. IEEE/ASME Trans Mechatr 17:136–146. https://doi.org/10.1109/TMECH.2010.2090353

Vaz DV, Silva PL, Mancini MC et al (2017) Towards an ecologically grounded functional practice in rehabilitation. Hum Mov Sci 52:117–132. https://doi.org/10.1016/j.humov.2017.01.010

Wakimoto S, Ogura K, Suzumori K, Nishioka Y (2009) Miniature soft hand with curling rubber pneumatic actuators. Proc IEEE Int Conf Robot Autom 14:556–561. https://doi.org/10.1109/ROBOT.2009.5152259

Wang Z, Polygerinos P, Overvelde JTB et al (2017a) Interaction forces of soft fiber reinforced bending actuators. IEEE/ASME Trans Mechatr 22:717–727. https://doi.org/10.1109/TMECH.2016.2638468

Wang B, McDaid A, Biglari-Abhari M, Aw KC (2017b) Design and development of a glove for post-stroke hand rehabilitation. In: Proceedings of the 2017 IEEE international conference on advanced intelligent mechatronics (AIM), pp 1047–1051

Winter J, Hunter S, Sim J, Crome P (2011) Hands-on therapy interventions for upper limb motor dysfunction following stroke. Cochrane Database Syst Rev 14:CD006609. https://doi.org/10.1002/14651858.CD006609.pub2

Worsnopp TT, Peshkin MA, Colgate JE, Kamper DG (2007) An actuated finger exoskeleton for hand rehabilitation following stroke. In: Proceedings of the 2007 IEEE 10th international conference on rehabilitation robotics, ICORR'07, pp 896–901

Yang J, Xie H, Shi J (2016) A novel motion-coupling design for a jointless tendon-driven finger exoskeleton for rehabilitation. Mech Mach Theory 99:83–102. https://doi.org/10.1016/j.mechmachtheory.2015.12.010

Yap HK, Lim JH, Nasrallah F et al (2015a) A soft exoskeleton for hand assistive and rehabilitation application using pneumatic actuators with variable stiffness. In: Proceedings of the 2015 IEEE international conference on robotics and automation (ICRA). IEEE, pp 4967–4972

Yap HK, Lim JH, Nasrallah F et al (2015b) MRC-glove: a fMRI compatible soft robotic glove for hand rehabilitation application. IEEE Int Confer Rehabil Robot 9:735–740. https://doi.org/10.1109/ICORR.2015.7281289

Yap HK, Goh JCH, Yeow RCH (2015c) Design and characterization of soft actuator for hand rehabilitation application. In: Lacković I, Vasic D (eds) Proceedings of European conference of the international federation for medical and biological engineering. Springer, Cham, pp 367–370

Yap HK, Ng HY, Yeow C-H (2016a) High-force soft printable pneumatics for soft robotic applications. Soft Robot 3:144–158. https://doi.org/10.1089/soro.2016.0030

Yap HK, Ang BWK, Lim JH et al (2016b) A fabric-regulated soft robotic glove with user intent detection using EMG and RFID for hand assistive application. Proc IEEE Int Conf Robot Autom 5:3537–3542. https://doi.org/10.1109/ICRA.2016.7487535

Yap HK, Lim JH, Nasrallah F et al (2017) Design and preliminary feasibility study of a soft robotic glove for hand function assistance in stroke survivors. Front Neurosci 11:1–14. https://doi.org/10.3389/fnins.2017.00547

Zhang J, Wang B, Zhang C et al (2019) An EEG/EMG/EOG-based multimodal human–machine interface to real-time control of a soft robot hand. Front Neurorobot 13:7. https://doi.org/10.3389/fnbot.2019.00007

Zhang Y, Wang D, Wang Z et al (2018) A two-fingered force feedback glove using soft actuators. In: Proceedings of the 2018 IEEE haptics symposium (HAPTICS), pp 186–191. https://doi.org/10.1109/HAPTICS.2018.8357174

Zhao H, Li Y, Elsamadisi A, Shepherd R (2015) Scalable manufacturing of high force wearable soft actuators. Extreme Mech Lett 3:89–104. https://doi.org/10.1016/j.eml.2015.02.006

Židek K, Boržíková J, Hošovský A et al (2012) Model-based evolution of a fast hybrid fuzzy adaptive controller for a pneumatic muscle actuator. Int J Adv Robot Syst 9:40. https://doi.org/10.5772/50347

Chapter 3
Bilateral Hand Rehabilitation Using a Soft Robotic Glove with Kinematics and EMG-Based Control

Soft hand exoskeletons are increasingly recognized as safer, lighter, and more affordable options for hand rehabilitation in hemiplegia patients compared to traditional rigid exoskeletons. This chapter introduces a soft robotic glove driven by a kinematics-EMG-based method, capable of replicating both the position and grasping force of the fingers in the unimpaired hand to the impaired hand of hemiplegic patients. A ten-degree-of-freedom bi-directional soft robotic glove was designed and characterized to enable patients to perform complex tasks and fine motor motions. An EMG-based method for estimating finger forces was developed and evaluated. Trajectory-following and grasping experiments demonstrated the system's effectiveness, with the robotic glove replicating the motion of the unimpaired hand with minimal delay (0.75 ± 0.34 s) and achieving a 68.8% success rate across various objects, with 96% success in grasping a regular bottle. These findings underscore the feasibility and potential of the system for bilateral hand rehabilitation in hemiplegic patients.

3.1 Introduction

Hemiplegia, commonly resulting from a stroke, causes a significant loss of motor function on a single side of the body, severely impacting daily living activities (ADLs) (Leonardis et al. 2015). A major contributor to hand dysfunction is weakness in finger muscles, particularly for finger extension (Cruz et al. 2005). Rehabilitation exercises targeting the impaired hand are crucial for restoring motor capacity. Robotic-assisted bilateral exercises have proven effective for improving rehabilitation outcomes in hemiplegic patients (Hesse et al. 2006, 2003; Li et al. 2009). For instance, Satoshi et al. developed an 18-degree-of-freedom (DOF) exoskeleton that facilitates bilateral hand training by mapping the healthy hand's joint positions to the impaired hand (Ueki et al. 2012). In our previous work, a data glove was utilized to capture the

M. Li and B. He, *Intention-Controlled Hand Rehabilitation for Stroke Survivors*,
https://doi.org/10.1007/978-981-95-4196-6_3

movement data of the intact hand, which was subsequently utilized to actuate a 3D-printed, pneumatically powered robotic glove (Li et al. 2020). This glove featured a design similar to the one presented in Chap. 2. However, both studies focused only on positional replication, not force transfer. Daniele et al. addressed this by creating a system that transfers the equivalent grasping force from the unimpaired to the impaired hand, but still lacks positional control (Leonardis et al. 2015). The integration of both position and force control in a rehabilitation system can enable more precise and functional hand motions.

Soft robotic exoskeletons, due to their lighter, safer, and more affordable nature, are emerging as a promising solution for rehabilitation (Aubin et al. 2013). Despite this, most existing soft exoskeletons focus on finger flexion assistance (Connelly et al. 2010; Yap et al. 2015), limiting the motion ability. To achieve more comprehensive rehabilitation, a system that enables bi-directional, multi-joint actuation is required. This chapter proposes a novel robotic-assisted bilateral hand rehabilitation system that uses a kinematics-EMG-based control method to simultaneously replicate both position and grasping force. The system, designed with a 10-DOF bi-directional soft robotic glove, allows for more complex and precise tasks. The glove's force estimation is based on EMG signals, enabling accurate control over both finger positions and forces during rehabilitation exercises.

The following sections detail the bilateral rehabilitation system design, soft robotic glove design, finger force estimation, kinematics and EMG-based control methods. We then present the experimental evaluation protocols and results, concluding with insights drawn from the validation studies.

3.2 Overall Design of the Bilateral Rehabilitation System

The rehabilitation system presented in this chapter consists of a soft robotic glove, a data glove, and a 4-channel EMG sensor. The soft robotic glove is worn on the affected hand to assist with its movement during rehabilitation exercises, while the data glove captures the kinematic information of the intact hand. The EMG sensor collects real-time signals from the forearm of the unimpaired hand.

Figure 3.1 illustrates the principle of the bilateral control method. The system operates by duplicating the unimpaired hand's motion and estimated grasping force onto the impaired hand when both hands interact with identical objects. Touch detection is first performed on each finger of the unimpaired hand. Before the finger touches the object, the soft robotic glove is controlled based on the kinematic data from the unimpaired hand. Once the finger makes contact with an object, the glove is controlled by the EMG signals from the unimpaired forearm. A multi-output artificial neural network (ANN) is employed to estimate the grasping force exerted by each finger in real-time. These estimated forces are then used as control signals to drive the soft robotic glove.

The mirror neuron system is thought to be activated through this process, facilitated by multiple sensory feedback channels (Leonardis et al. 2015). This combined

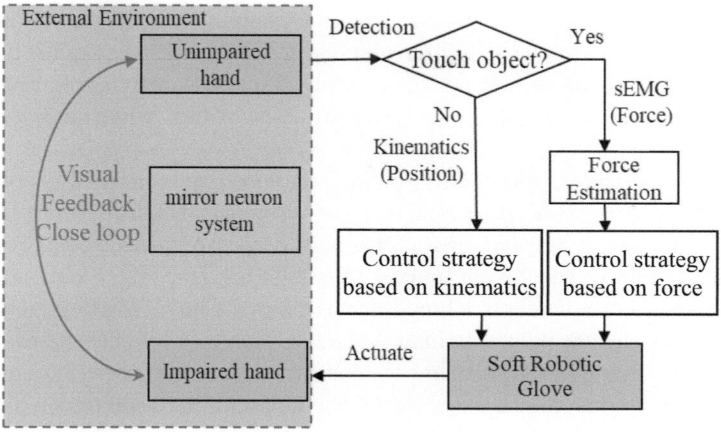

Fig. 3.1 Sketch of the control method based on kinematics and EMG

approach—using both kinematic and force feedback—enables patients to perform more complex and fine motor tasks than systems relying solely on force (Leonardis et al. 2015) or position control (Ueki et al. 2012).

3.3 Soft Robotic Glove Design and Fabrication

Both the design and fabrication of the soft robotic glove for bilateral hand rehabilitation are crucial for achieving both effective and precise movements while maintaining system simplicity. The glove features a total of 10 DOFs, balancing the need for complex control with the goal of maintaining an efficient rehabilitation process. The actuators for the proximal interphalangeal (PIP) joint and distal interphalangeal (DIP) joint in each finger are combined into a single DOF, as these joints typically move in concert. Therefore, each finger actuator consists of two DOFs, corresponding to the movement of the metacarpophalangeal (MCP) joint and the combined PIP/DIP joints.

To keep the overall weight of the glove manageable, it was designed to weigh <0.5 kg, ensuring comfort and practicality for prolonged use in rehabilitation exercises (Zhou et al. 2019).

Each joint's range of motion (ROM) in the glove was designed according to standard clinical guidelines, as outlined by Hume et al. (1990). The normal ROM for the thumb's MCP joint, interphalangeal (IPJ) joint, the MCP joint of the other four fingers, and the sum ROM for the PIP/DIP joints of the four fingers are 56°, 78°, 100°, and 190°, respectively. For stroke patients, the motion range is typically limited to about two-thirds of the normal range to avoid overextension and strain (Ma and Ruan 2022). As a result, the actuators are designed to bend at two-thirds of the typical range of each joint.

For optimal grasping functionality, the glove's output force must be sufficient to grasp typical objects in our daily life, which generally weigh <1.5 kg (Polygerinos et al. 2015). Based on this, the glove's output force was designed to exceed 7.3 N (Polygerinos et al. 2015), ensuring it can assist with a wide range of object manipulations.

Pneumatic actuators, particularly folding structures, are commonly used in soft robotic gloves for their efficiency and flexibility (Keong and Hua 2018). As shown in Figs. 3.2 and 3.3, in our design, two air channels are used to provide both flexion and extension assistance. The flexion actuator inflates to bend the finger joints, while the extension actuator provides stretching force to return the finger to a neutral position.

The flexion actuator inflates to induce bending motion, while the extension actuator stretches the finger. To account for the fact that finger extension angles are generally smaller than the bending angles, the height of the bending air channel is designed to be less than that of the extension part.

As shown in Fig. 3.3, the actuators were manufactured using a 3D printer (Raise3D E2, Shanghai Fuzhi Information Technology Co., Ltd, China) with NinjaFlex 85A

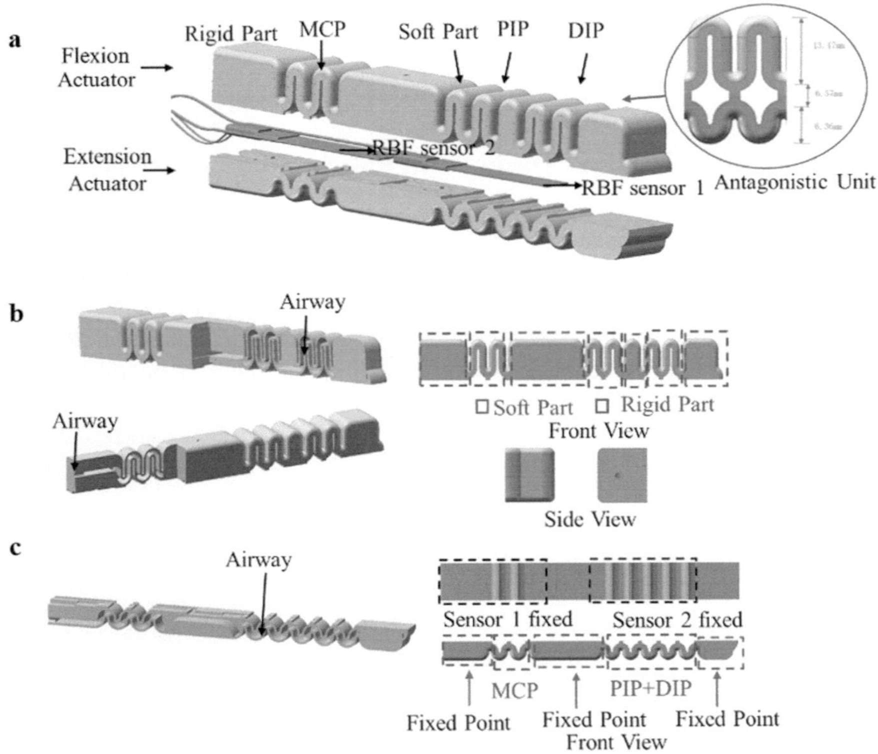

Fig. 3.2 The design of the finger actuator: **a** 3D view, **b** flexion part, and **c** extension part

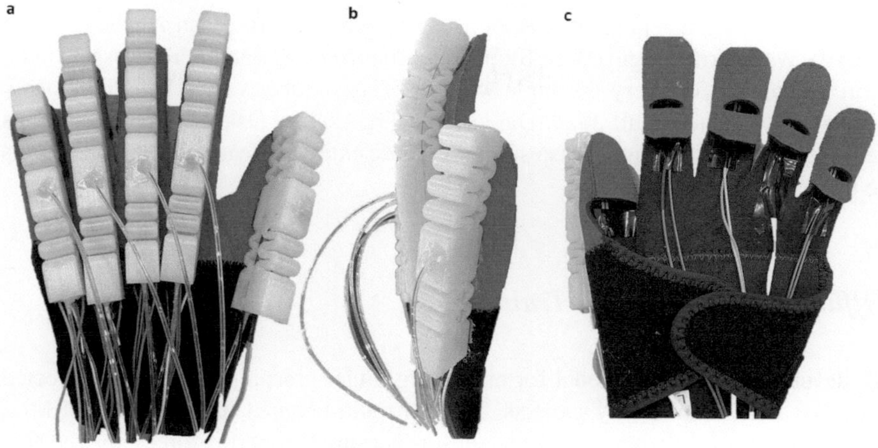

Fig. 3.3 Prototype of the soft robotic glove

material. Angle sensors were embedded between the flexion and extension components to accurately monitor joint movements. A commercial fabric glove was used to attach the actuators to the patient's hand, ensuring comfort and ease of use.

3.4 Finger Force Estimation Based on EMG Signal

This section describes the method utilized to measure the individual finger force during grasping based on EMG signals from the unimpaired forearm.

Data Preprocessing

EMG signals were collected using an EMG sensor (NeuSen WM, Neuracle, China) and underwent the following preprocessing steps:

- Moving Window and Filtering: A moving window of m samples was applied to the EMG data, which was then processed using a sixth-order Butterworth lowpass filter to remove motion artifacts.
- Frequency Interference Removal: A notch filter set at 50 Hz was used to eliminate electrical noise from the power line.
- Bandpass Filtering: A bandpass filter extracted the characteristic frequency bands of the EMG signal.
- Envelope Extraction: The Hilbert transform was applied to extract the envelope of the filtered signal.

Next, the parameters include Root Mean Square (RMS), Mean Absolute Value (MAV), Waveform Length (WL), Slope Sign Change (SSC), and Zero Crossing (ZC) were calculated for every n-sample window. These features have been previously validated (Martinez et al. 2020; Dai et al. 2017; Asghari Oskoei and Hu 2007) as reliable indicators of finger grasp strength. These extracted features served as inputs to the neural network model.

Offline Neural Network Training

To develop a prediction model for estimating finger grasping forces, we collected a dataset from four healthy subjects. The raw multi-channel surface EMG (sEMG) signals were used as input, and the sensor-measured fingertip forces for the five fingers served as output labels. As sEMG signals are inherently non-stationery and time-varying, we recorded EMG data at a sampling rate of 1000 Hz from different subjects to improve the model's generalizability.

In the training process, firstly, subjects were asked to gradually increase their grip force along the contact surface between their finger and the force sensor. The force should rise smoothly from the baseline to a peak (within 2 s), be maintained at peak force for 2 s, and then decrease back to baseline within another 2 s. Each trial included three target force levels (~2, 5, and 10 N) and was repeated 24 times per subject, with 10-s rest periods between trials.

A backpropagation (BP) neural network was used to model the nonlinear relationship between muscular activity (sEMG) and the corresponding grasping force. The network architecture comprised three layers: an input layer containing 20 nodes (corresponding to the 20 extracted features), a hidden layer containing 128 nodes, and an output layer consisting of 5 nodes, each corresponding to one of the five fingers' forces. The activation function of the hidden layer was the sigmoid function, mapping the output to the range (0, 1). The training was performed using mini-batch optimization. The weights were updated via backpropagation.

The weight matrix from input to hidden layer was $\omega_{ij}^{(1)}$. Hidden-to-output weights was set in $\omega_{ij}^{(2)}$. The output force vector was $f = [f_1, f_2, f_3, f_4, f_5]$. The mathematical formulation of the neural network is presented below:

$$h_j^{(1)} = \text{Sigmoid}\left(\sum_{i=0} w_{ij}^{(1)} * x_i\right) \tag{3.1}$$

$$f_k = \sum_{j=0} w_i^{(2)} h_j \tag{3.2}$$

where x_i is the ith input node, and f_k is the kth output node.

The loss function is formulated as the mean squared error between the predicted and actual force:

Table 3.1 Hyperparameters selection

Parameters	Search space	Selected value
Batch size	32, 64, 128, 256	128
Learning rate	0.0001, 0.001, 0.005, 0.01	0.01
Number of hidden nodes	16, 32, 64, 128	128
Epoch count	100, 500, 1000	1000

$$\text{Error} = \frac{1}{N}\sum_{n=1}^{N}(f_{kn} - y_{kn})^2 \tag{3.3}$$

where N is the batch size, f_{kn} is the predicted output value, and y_{kn} is the label.

Hyperparameters such as learning rate, batch size, epoch count, and the number of hidden layer neurons were tuned using fourfold cross-validation to optimize model performance. Early stopping was employed to prevent overfitting. The optimal hyperparameters, selected after testing various configurations, are summarized in Table 3.1.

3.5 Kinematics and EMG-Based Control Method

The kinematics-EMG-based control method combines both kinematic data and estimated finger forces to control the movement of the robotic glove. The algorithm is summarized in Table 3.2. Parameters are calculated by using Eqs. (3.4)–(3.12). The meanings of the used symbols are shown in Table 3.3.

$$\delta = f_{\text{tip}_i} - f_{0_i} \tag{3.4}$$

$$\text{Sig}_1\left(f_{\text{tip}_i}\right) = \begin{cases} 1, & |\delta| < \xi \\ 0, & |\delta| \geq \xi \end{cases} \tag{3.5}$$

$$\text{Sig}_2\left(f_{\text{tip}_i}\right) = \begin{cases} 1, & |\delta| \geq \xi \\ 0, & |\delta| < \xi \end{cases} \tag{3.6}$$

$$p_{ij} = \text{Sig}_1\left(f_{\text{tip}_i}\right)p_{0_{ij}} + \text{Sig}_2\left(f_{\text{tip}_i}\right)\Delta p_{ij} \tag{3.7}$$

$$q_{ij} = k * p_{ij} \tag{3.8}$$

$$\Phi_{ij} = \begin{bmatrix} A_{ij} & B_{ij} & C_{ij} \end{bmatrix} \begin{bmatrix} \alpha_{ij}^2 \\ \alpha_{ij} \\ 1 \end{bmatrix} \tag{3.9}$$

$$\Psi_{ij} = \begin{bmatrix} M_{ij} & N_{ij} \end{bmatrix} \begin{bmatrix} g_i & g_i \\ 1 & 1 \end{bmatrix} \tag{3.10}$$

$$p_{0_{ij}} = \Phi_{ij} + \varepsilon \tag{3.11}$$

$$\Delta p_{ij} = \Psi_{ij} + \eta \tag{3.12}$$

Figure 3.4 illustrates the overall control framework, where the flow of information between the modules is as follows:

- The kinematic data and raw EMG signals from the unimpaired hand are processed and converted into corresponding digital values.
- These values are sent to analog input/output modules and subsequently used to control the output pressure of the electromagnetic proportional valves (IVT0030-2BL, SMC, Japan).
- An air compressor (S1600W-30L, AOTUSI, China) supplies the air source for the actuators.
- The actuators' movements are monitored by embedded angle sensors (RFP, Yutong Technology Co., LTD, China), while contact forces on the impaired hand are measured by force sensors (Fingertips, Pressure Profile Systems, Los Angeles, CA, USA).

Table 3.2 Kinematics and EMG-based control algorithm

	Input: α_{ij}, s_t
	Output: q_{ij}, $p_{0_{ij}}$
1	Initialize A, B, C, M, N
2	s_t was high pass filtered (6th-order Butterworth, $f_c = 15$ Hz), notch filtered at the power-line frequency (5th-order Butterworth at 50 Hz, notch bandwidth of 3 Hz), bandpass filtered (6th-order Butterworth, $f_{c1} = 17.5, f_{c2} = 482.5$Hz), Hilbert transformed, and feature extracted. (RMS, MAV, WL, ZC, SSC)
3	Derive estimated reference force using Neural network: $g_1, g_2, \ldots, g_5$
4	If $\lvert\delta\rvert \geq \xi$ then
	Derive kinematics-controlled pressure $p_{ij} = \Delta p_{1,1}, \Delta p_{1,2}, \ldots \Delta p_{5,2}$
	Else derive kinematics-controlled pressure@ @$p_{ij} = p_{0_{11}}, p_{0_{12}}, \ldots p_{0_{52}}$
	End if
5	If $p_{0_{ij}} \leq q_{ij} \leq q_{\text{boundary}}$ then
	Output q_{ij}@ @Else output $p_{0_{ij}}$ @ @end if

Table 3.3 Nomenclature

Abbreviation	Meanings of each abbreviation
p_{ij}	Pressure of the *j*th joint of the *i*th finger
α_{ij}	Bending angle of the *j*th joint of the *i*th finger
q_{ij}	Control voltage of the *j*th joint of the *i*th finger
q_{boundary}	Control voltage boundary
$p_{0_{ij}}$	Kinematics-controlled pressure
Δp_{ij}	EMG-controlled pressure
ε	Error of kinematics-controlled pressure
η	Error of EMG-controlled pressure
g_i	Estimated grasping force of the *i*th finger
Φ	Kinematics-controlled pressure generation model
ψ	EMG-controlled pressure generation model
k	Proportional coefficient of valves
f_{tip_i}	Contact force of the *i*th finger
δ	Given contact force threshold
ξ	Trigger threshold of fingertip contact force
A, B, C	Transfer function matrix of kinematics
M, N	Transfer function matrix of grasping force

3.6 Experimental Protocol

Evaluation of the Proposed Finger Force Estimation Method

This section evaluates the performance of the finger force estimation model. Four healthy subjects (right-handed, aged 20–24 years, male) were recruited. The maximum voluntary contraction (MVC) was tested for each subject to normalize the EMG and force data. The force amplitude increased from baseline to peak within 3–4 s, remained at peak for 2 s, and then decreased to zero over 2 s. This process was repeated three times, with 2-min rest intervals between each trial. Follow-up tests were only conducted when the maximum force difference between two consecutive trials did not exceed 5%. A 400 ms window centered on the peak force was selected for MVC calculation. The RMES and R^2 values between the real and estimated forces were used to evaluate the model's performance. This research received ethical approval from the Institutional Review Board of Xi'an Jiaotong University.

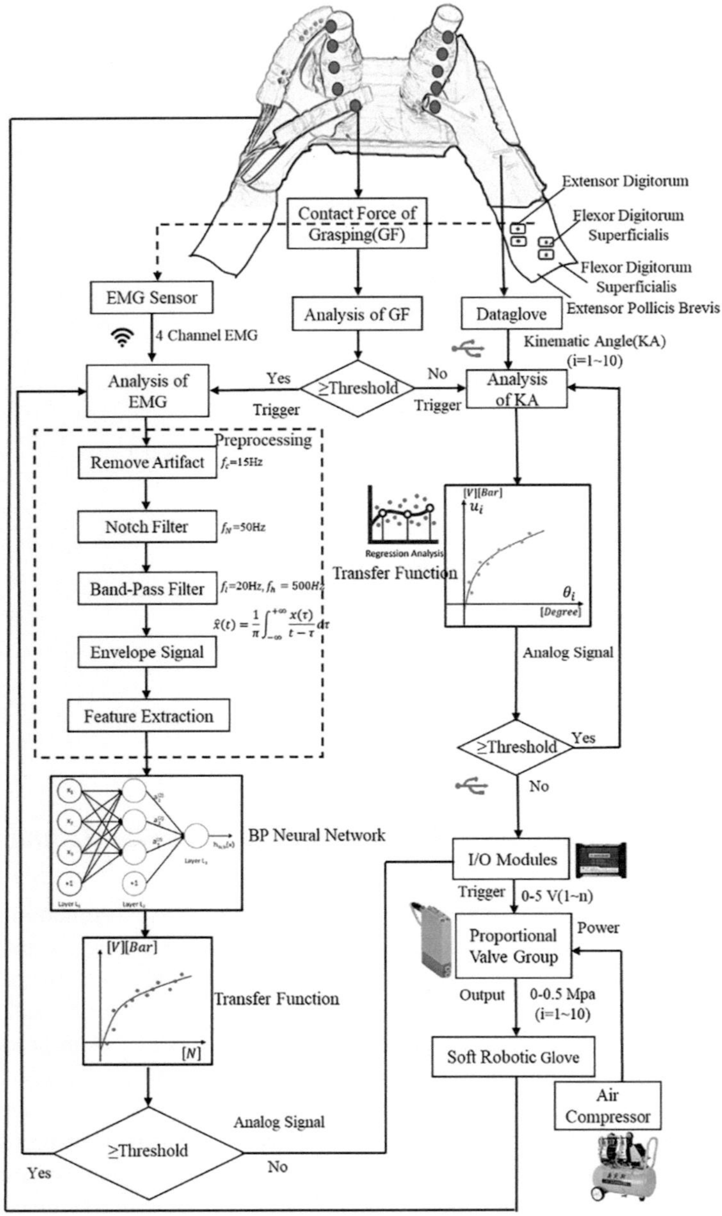

Fig. 3.4 Details of the whole control framework

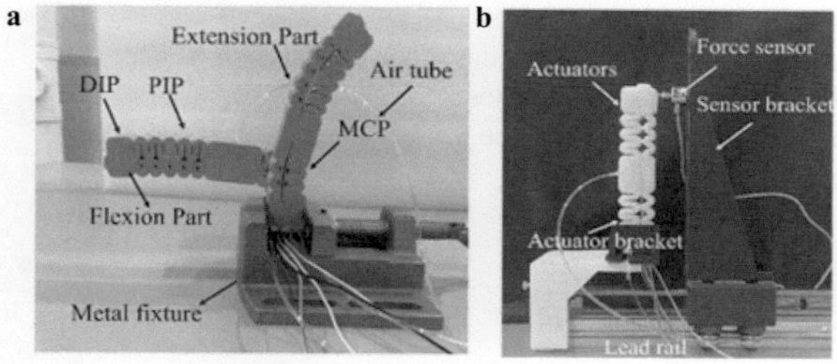

Fig. 3.5 **a** ROM testing platform. **b** Output force testing platform

Characterization for Actuators of the Soft Robotic Glove

Experiments were conducted to validate the ROM and output force performance of the actuators in the soft robotic glove (see Fig. 3.5). In the ROM test, the deformation behavior of the actuators was investigated at various inflation pressure levels (ranging from 0.05 to 0.5 MPa, with 0.05 MPa intervals). A digital camera captured the angle changes of the actuators, and a specialized toolbox in Photoshop CS6 (Adobe, USA) was used to calculate the actuator angles. In the output force test, the force produced by the actuator was recorded using a calibrated force sensor (BSLM-1, Bufson Sensor, CN) with 16-bit resolution. The output force was measured as the pressure was gradually applied to the flexion actuator, reaching up to 0.3 MPa. Five trials were repeated for each pressure setting.

Relationship Between Driven Voltage and Output Force of Pneumatic Actuators

To accurately control the soft robotic glove actuators and generate the target force, the correlation between the output force and the driving voltage of the pneumatic actuators was investigated. A healthy subject wore the soft robotic glove and fingertip force measurement sensors, as shown in Fig. 3.6. First, the subject was asked to adjust their fingers to ensure a stable grasping force before starting the experiment. The pneumatic actuators' inner pressure was varied between 0.5 and 4 MPa, with intervals of 0.5 MPa. Simultaneously, the force and driving voltage were recorded. The experiment was repeated for each finger with eight trials per condition. Figure 3.6 illustrates the experimental platform used to estimate the individual finger force based on the driven voltage of the pneumatic actuators.

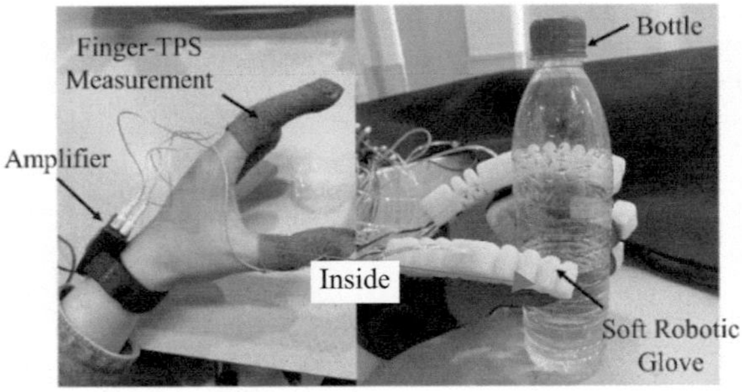

Fig. 3.6 The experimental platform used to estimate the individual finger force based on the driven voltage of the pneumatic actuators

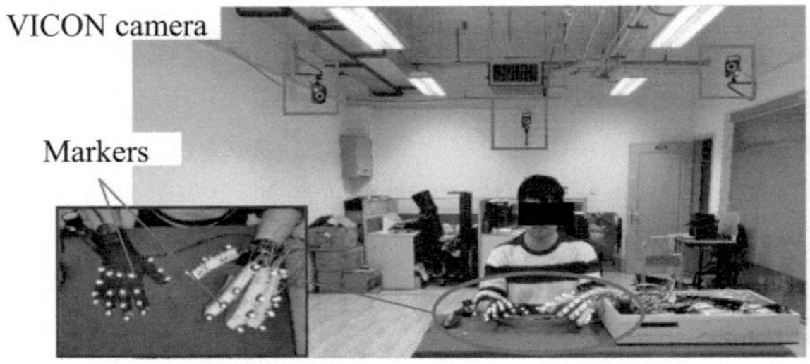

Fig. 3.7 Experimental platform for joint angle measurement by the VICON T40S capture system

Evaluation of Bilateral Motion Control

To validate the feasibility of the kinematics-based bilateral motion control, one subject was involved in this experiment. The subject was instructed to move their hands with the assistance of the glove. In this experiment, the subject's left hand (designated as the impaired hand) was relaxed, while the right hand (designated as the unimpaired hand) moved naturally. Figure 3.7 shows the VICON T40s motion capture system used to record the joint angles of both hands at a frame rate of 500 frames per second (OML Co., UK). The captured position data of the markers were processed to calculate the joint angles, providing a detailed measurement of hand motion during the experiment.

Evaluation of Bilateral Grasping Control

To evaluate the effectiveness of the system for bilateral grasping, an object grasping experiment was conducted (see Fig. 3.8). A soft robotic glove was worn on the left hand (representing the impaired hand), and a data glove (WiseGlove 14, Xintian-shijing Technology, China) with muscle electrodes was worn on the right hand and forearm. The left hand was completely relaxed, while the right hand controlled the left hand's grasping through the proposed kinematics and EMG-based control method. The experiment involved 15 objects of varying sizes and weights, including wooden

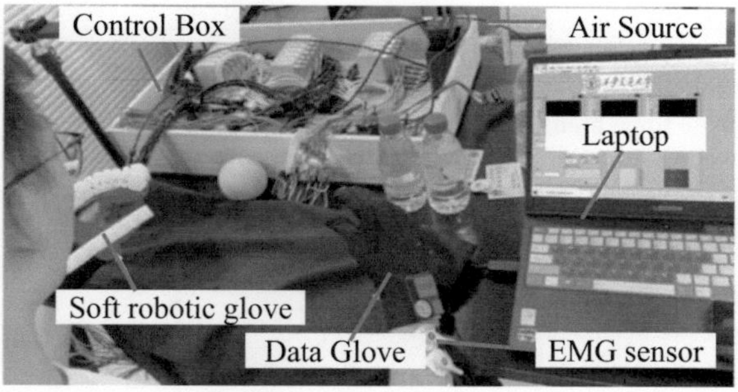

Fig. 3.8 Object grasping experiment setup

ball, thermos cup, water bottles (550, 250, 125 g), marker pen, tennis ball, mouse, eraser, tape rolls, landmines model, silicone bottle, empty bottle, and stylus. The subjects were instructed to use their right hand to control their left hand and grasp the objects. After successfully grasping an object, they were asked to hold it for 4 s and then return it to its original position. The time taken from the initiation of the movement of the right hand to the return of the left hand to the rest position was recorded. Five trials were performed for each object.

3.7 Experimental Results

Force Estimation Results

The experimental results of one representative subject are shown in Fig. 3.9. The upper panels compare the estimated grasping force (from the neural network output) with the measured force of five fingers (reference from the neural network). These comparisons demonstrate relatively good tracking performance. The lower panels show linear regression results between the estimated and measured forces. The correlation coefficients (R^2) for the five fingers from thumb to little finger are 0.94, 0.89, 0.95, 0.93, and 0.78, respectively, with biases of 0.13, 0.27, 0.17, 0.14, and 0.08. These results suggest good accuracy in the force estimation method.

Table 3.4 summarizes the Mean Absolute Error (MAE), R^2, and bias (b) for each subject. In ideal conditions (Subjects 3 and 4), R^2 is close to 1 and the bias is near 0.1. The maximum force estimation error across subjects was 8.85%, indicating that the method is robust across different users.

Performance of the Bidirectional Soft Robotic Glove

Figure 3.10 illustrates the motion range of the actuators. At 0.5 MPa, the maximum bending angles for the MCP joints of the five fingers from thumb to little fingers

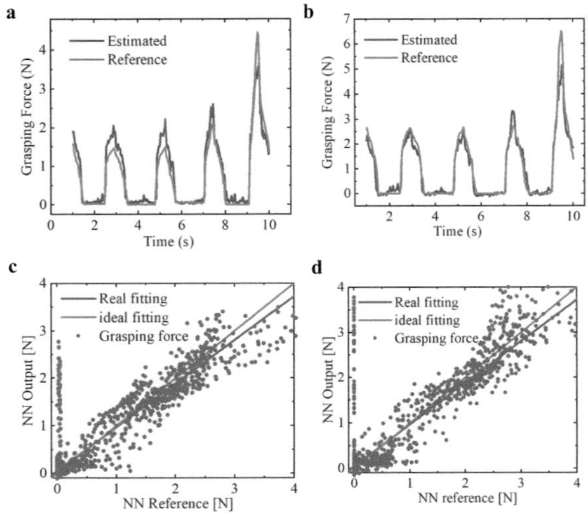

Fig. 3.9 Force estimation results. **a** The force monitoring for the thumb, **b** the force monitoring for the index finger, **c** the relationship between the predicted and benchmark forces for the thumb, and **d** the relationship between the predicted and benchmark forces for the index finger

Table 3.4 Performance of Force Estimation

Subjects	Fingers	MAE (MVC%)	R^2	*B* (Bias) [N]
Subject 1	Thumb	2.78	0.58	0.10
	Index	8.07	0.48	0.58
	Middle	5.22	0.42	0.35
	Ring	3.07	0.51	0.23
	Pinky	2.47	0.58	0.18
Subject 2	Thumb	1.78	0.81	0.05
	Index	3.84	0.80	0.19
	Middle	5.09	0.80	0.11
	Ring	8.85	0.78	0.26
	Pinky	6.50	0.77	0.13
Subject 3	Thumb	2.65	0.92	0.09
	Index	3.89	0.92	0.08
	Middle	3.57	0.95	0.11
	Ring	3.27	0.96	0.15
	Pinky	2.47	0.93	0.13
Subject 4	Thumb	3.05	0.94	0.13
	Index	7.89	0.89	0.27
	Middle	3.27	0.95	0.17
	Ring	2.85	0.93	0.14
	Pinky	8.50	0.78	-0.08

were 95.13°, 97.17°, 84.47°, 87°, and 91.47°, respectively. The sum of the motion angles for the PIP and DIP joints for the index, middle, ring, and pinky were 176.57°, 160.6°, 163.63°, and 124.97°, respectively. The bending angle for the thumb's IP joint was 130.63°. The actuators' maximum extension angles exceeded 40°, indicating sufficient ROM for ADLs and finger rehabilitation.

In Fig. 3.10f, the maximum output forces were 4.45 (thumb), 4.36 (index), 5.62 (middle), 5.08 (ring), and 5.22 N (pinky). The total output force for all five fingers was 24.7 ± 0.74 N, which meets the requirements for ADL assistance as outlined in Sect. 3.3.

Relationship Between the Driving Voltage and the Actuator's Output Force

The relationship between the driving voltage and grasping force for each finger is shown in Fig. 3.11a. The maximum grasping forces were 4.63 N (thumb), 3.27 N (index), 3.74 N (middle), 3.74 N (ring), and 4.54 N (pinky). The relationship between the driving voltage (U) and grasping force (F) is summarized in Table 3.5, which can be used for precise control of the actuators during bilateral rehabilitation.

Results of Bilateral Motion Control

As shown in Fig. 3.11b, the trajectory of the impaired hand, assisted by the soft robotic glove, closely followed the reference trajectory generated by the unimpaired hand. However, errors were observed when the reference angle changed rapidly due to the limited driving voltage. Table 3.6 shows the relative standard errors for the joint angles of the impaired hand. Additionally, a noticeable hysteresis was observed in the joint motion of the unimpaired hand due to inherent system response delays. The average delay was 0.75 ± 0.34 s.

Performance of Bilateral Grasping

The grasping duration and success rates for the 15 objects are shown in Fig. 3.12. The average grasping time across all objects was 11.39 ± 2.8 s. The time to grasp moderately sized objects (e.g., thermos cups) was shorter than for smaller or irregularly shaped objects (e.g., mouse). The average grasping success rate was 68.8%, with the lowest being 48% for the mouse and the highest being 96% for the silicone bottle.

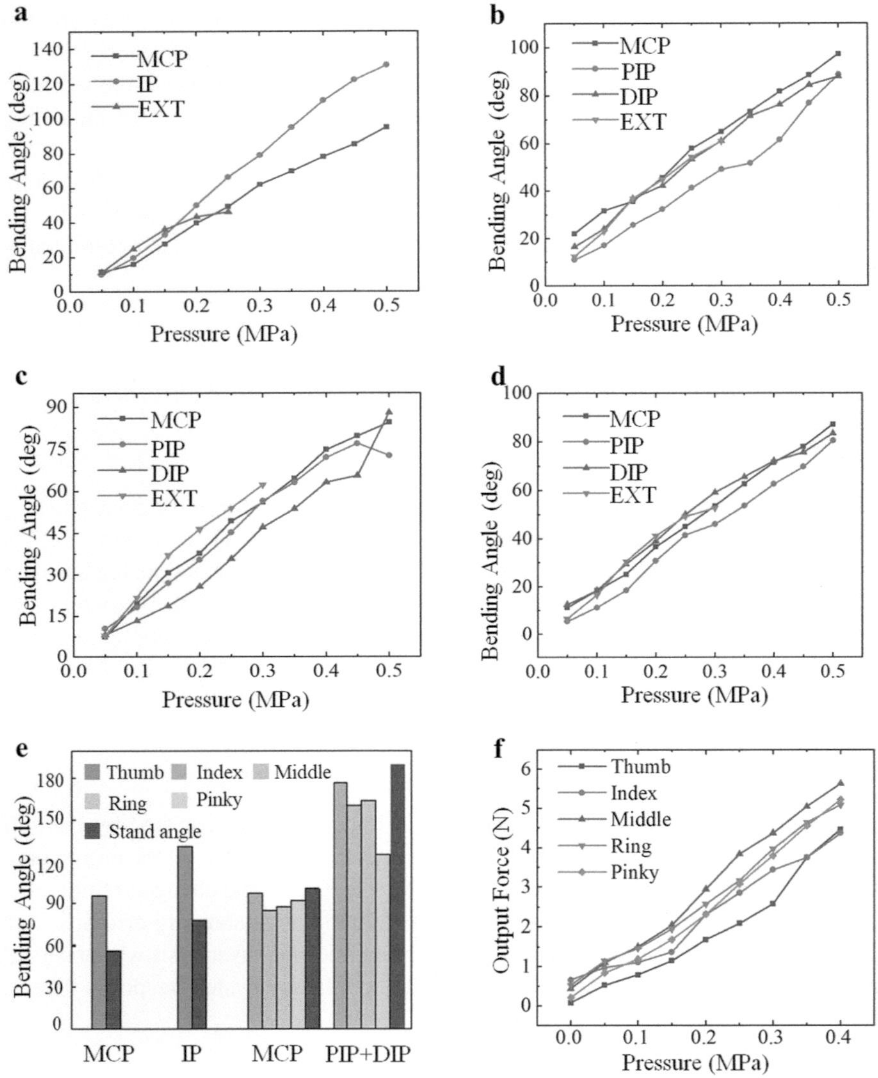

Fig. 3.10 Characterization results for the bidirectional soft robotic glove. **a–d** Motion range of the actuators corresponding to the thumb, index, middle, and ring finger, respectively. EXT is the extension angle. **e** Comparison between the bending angles of actuators corresponding to finger joints and the stand angles. The stand angles are the motion range of the hand joint measured in [29]. PIP + DIP means the motion range of the actuator corresponding to the PIP and the DIP. **f** The output force of the thumb, index, middle, ring, and pinky, respectively

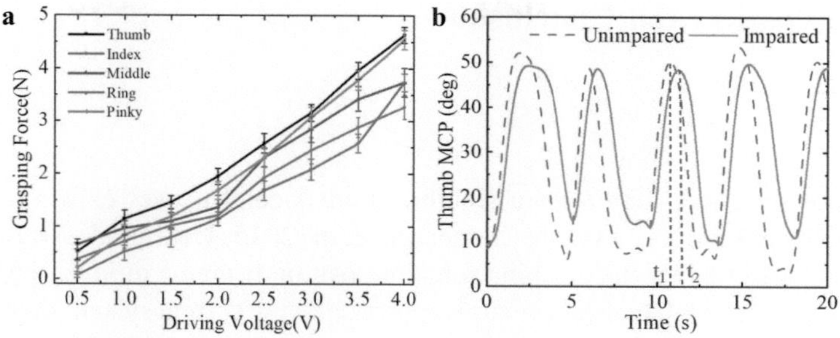

Fig. 3.11 **a** Quantitative estimation result between driving voltage and grasping force. **b** MCP joint angle responses of impaired and unimpaired hands in self-motion control

Table 3.5 Relationship between the driving voltage and grasping force

Fingers	Relationship
Thumb	U = 0.879F-0.071
Index	U = 0.806F + 0.335
Middle	U = 0.872F + 0.0234
Ring	U = 0.838F + 0.054
Pinky	U = 0.862F + 0.022

Table 3.6 Relative standard error of the impaired hand joint

Fingers	MCP (%)	PIP (%)	DIP (%)
Thumb	9.70	8.36	\
Index	9.79	9.87	10.85
Middle	8.82	10.48	9.77
Ring	8.48	10.34	9.78
Pinky	7.04	6.85	9.19

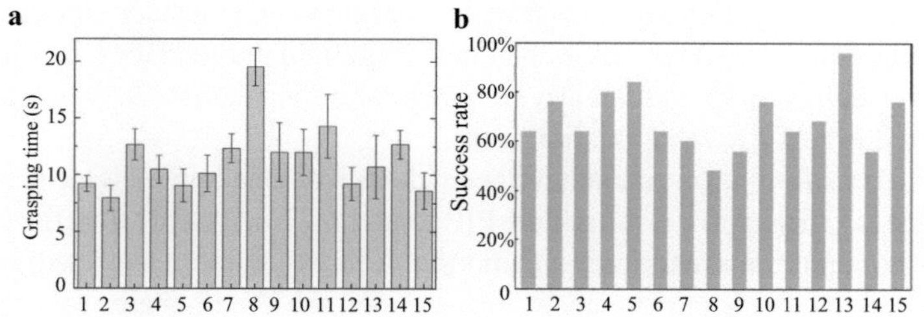

Fig. 3.12 Experimental results of grasping 15 objects assisted by exoskeleton. These objects in order are a wooden ball, a thermos cup, a water bottle A (550 g), a water bottle B (250 g), a water bottle C (125 g), a marker pen, a tennis ball, a mouse, an eraser, a small tape, a large tape, a landmines model, a bottle for silicone, an empty bottle, and a stylus. **a** The amount of time it takes to complete different object grasping, and **b** average success rate of grasping objects

3.8 Discussion and Conclusion

Discussion

The proposed system represents a significant advancement over existing robotic-assisted bilateral training systems (Leonardis et al. 2015; Ueki et al. 2012), which primarily transfer either the grasping force or position from the unimpaired hand to the impaired hand. Unlike these previous approaches, the current system successfully reproduces both the position and the grasping force of the unimpaired hand, offering more comprehensive assistance for rehabilitation. This dual transfer of both position and force could potentially enhance the rehabilitation outcomes for stroke patients by providing more natural and intuitive movement assistance. However, further studies are required to directly compare the efficacy of this method with other approaches, such as those proposed by Chen et al. (2023), where foot movements are used to control the hand/forearm exoskeleton. A comparative analysis of these systems would help identify the most effective control strategies and the specific advantages of each.

In terms of hardware performance, the actuators used in the proposed system successfully meet the necessary bending angle and force output requirements, ensuring adequate assistance for bilateral rehabilitation tasks. The lightweight design of the glove (weighing only 0.144 kg) is another important achievement, as it significantly reduces the strain on the user compared to previous designs that often exceeded 0.5 kg. This makes the system more practical for prolonged use during daily rehabilitation training, contributing to improved patient compliance and comfort.

The grasping control experiments demonstrate promising results, with high success rates for grasping common objects. For example, the system achieved an 84% success rate for a 125 g water bottle and a 96% success rate for a silicone bottle. However, the system's performance was less reliable for objects with irregular shapes, such as a computer mouse, where grasping time increased and success rates decreased. Additionally, the system struggled with heavier objects, which further reduced performance. These challenges highlight the need for future improvements in object handling, particularly for irregular or heavier items, which are often encountered in real-life rehabilitation tasks.

Several areas for improvement have been identified. One critical issue is potential actuator leaks, particularly in the middle PIP actuator, which could affect the system's ability to maintain consistent force and motion. Addressing these leaks will be essential for ensuring reliable performance over extended use. Another area for refinement is the system's response delay. While the current design is functional, further reducing the delay between user input and system response would enhance the overall user experience and boost the system's effectiveness in real-time rehabilitation scenarios.

Looking ahead, future experiments could explore the integration of humanoid robotic hands instead of human hands to provide more accurate measurements of motion and force assistance. This would allow for more precise quantification of the system's capabilities and better performance evaluation. Additionally, the use of humanoid hands might offer greater flexibility in testing a wider range of object types and sizes, further improving the system's robustness.

To summarize, while the proposed system shows considerable promise in supporting bilateral rehabilitation, ongoing refinements are necessary to address actuator performance, response delays, and object handling capabilities. With these improvements, the system could become a more effective tool for assisting stroke survivors in regaining functional independence.

Conclusion

In this chapter, we presented a robotic-assisted bilateral hand rehabilitation system that integrates both kinematics- and EMG-based control methods. This innovative system can replicate both the position and grasping force of the unimpaired hand onto the impaired hand, offering more comprehensive assistance during rehabilitation. The soft robotic glove, equipped with bi-directional, multi-joint actuation, effectively supports bilateral rehabilitation training, while a novel EMG-based finger force estimation method enhances the system's responsiveness to user intentions.

Experimental results demonstrate that the actuators in the soft robotic glove meet the clinical requirements for bending angles and output force. The bilateral motion control experiment showed a maximum trajectory error of 10.85% across all finger joints, with an average response delay of 0.75 ± 0.34 s. Grasping experiments revealed that the average time for performing a rehabilitation grasp motion was 11.39 ± 2.8 s, including a 4-s hold, with an overall success rate of 68.8%. The highest success rate of 96% was achieved when grasping a silicone bottle, highlighting the system's potential for assisting in everyday tasks. Furthermore, the glove's lightweight design (0.144 kg) significantly reduces the burden on the user's hand, enhancing comfort and usability during extended training sessions.

For future work, we aim to develop a more advanced, unsupervised force estimation method that could further refine the system's performance. Additionally, we plan to optimize the bi-directional, multi-joint actuators to minimize trajectory discrepancies between the impaired and unimpaired hands. Future studies will also involve participants with specific conditions, such as individuals with a history of hemiplegia, to assess the system's applicability across a broader range of clinical populations.

Overall, this system represents a significant step forward in the field of robotic-assisted rehabilitation, with promising potential for enhancing the effectiveness of bilateral hand rehabilitation, particularly for individuals recovering from stroke and other motor impairments.

References

Asghari-Oskoei M, Hu H (2007) Myoelectric control systems: a survey. Biomed Sig Process Control 2:275–294. https://doi.org/10.1016/j.bspc.2007.07.009

Aubin PM, Sallum H, Walsh C et al (2013) A pediatric robotic thumb exoskeleton for at-home rehabilitation: the isolated orthosis for thumb actuation (IOTA). In: IEEE international conference on rehabilitation robotics. https://doi.org/10.1109/ICORR.2013.6650500

Chen W, Li G, Li N et al (2023) Restoring voluntary bimanual activities of patients with chronic hemiparesis through a foot-controlled hand/forearm exoskeleton. IEEE Trans Neural Syst Rehabil Eng 31:769–778. https://doi.org/10.1109/TNSRE.2022.3233631

Connelly L, Jia Y, Toro ML et al (2010) A pneumatic glove and immersive virtual reality environment for hand rehabilitative training after stroke. IEEE Trans Neural Syst Rehabil Eng 18:551–559. https://doi.org/10.1109/TNSRE.2010.2047588

Cruz EG, Waldinger HC, Kamper DG (2005) Kinetic and kinematic workspaces of the index finger following stroke. Brain 128:1112–1121. https://doi.org/10.1093/brain/awh432

Dai C, Bardizbanian B, Clancy EA (2017) Comparison of constant-posture force-varying EMG-force dynamic models about the elbow. IEEE Trans Neural Syst Rehabil Eng 25:1529–1538. https://doi.org/10.1109/TNSRE.2016.2639443

Hesse S, Schulte-Tigges G, Konrad M et al (2003) Robot-assisted arm trainer for the passive and active practice of bilateral forearm and wrist movements in hemiparetic subjects. Arch Phys Med Rehabil 84:915–920. https://doi.org/10.1016/S0003-9993(02)04954-7

Hesse S, Schmidt H, Werner C (2006) Machines to support motor rehabilitation after stroke: 10 years of experience in Berlin. J Rehabil Res Dev 43:671–678. https://doi.org/10.1682/JRRD.2005.02.0052

Hume MC, Gellman H, McKellop H, Brumfield RH (1990) Functional range of motion of the joints of the hand. J Hand Surg Am 15:240–243. https://doi.org/10.1016/0363-5023(90)90102-W

Keong BAW, Hua RYC (2018) A novel fold-based design approach toward printable soft robotics using flexible 3D printing materials. Adv Mater Technol 3:1700172. https://doi.org/10.1002/admt.201700172

Leonardis D, Barsotti M, Loconsole C et al (2015) An EMG-controlled robotic hand exoskeleton for bilateral rehabilitation. IEEE Trans Hapt 8:140–151. https://doi.org/10.1109/TOH.2015.2417570

Li S, Frisoli A, Avizzano CA et al (2009) Bimanual haptic-desktop platform for upper-limb post-stroke rehabilitation: Practical trials. In: Proceedings of the 2009 IEEE international conference on robotics and biomimetics, ROBIO 2009, pp 480–485. https://doi.org/10.1109/ROBIO.2009.5420694

Li M, Wang T, Zhuo Y et al (2020) A soft robotic glove for hand rehabilitation training controlled by movements of the healthy hand. In: Proceedings of the 2020 17th international conference on ubiquitous robots, UR 2020

Ma J, Ruan X (2022) Application effect of early comprehensive rehabilitation nursing in patients with acute ischemic stroke. Clin Res Pract 7:176–178

Martinez IJR, Mannini A, Clemente F, Cipriani C (2020) Online grasp force estimation from the transient EMG. IEEE Trans Neural Syst Rehabil Eng 28:2333–2341. https://doi.org/10.1109/TNSRE.2020.3022587

Polygerinos P, Wang Z, Galloway KC et al (2015) Soft robotic glove for combined assistance and at-home rehabilitation. Rob Auton Syst 73:135–143. https://doi.org/10.1016/j.robot.2014.08.014

Ueki S, Kawasaki H, Ito S et al (2012) Development of a hand-assist robot with multi-degrees-of-freedom for rehabilitation therapy. IEEE/ASME Trans Mechatr 17:136–146. https://doi.org/10.1109/TMECH.2010.2090353

Yap HK, Lim JH, Nasrallah F et al (2015) A soft exoskeleton for hand assistive and rehabilitation application using pneumatic actuators with variable stiffness. Proc IEEE Int Conf Robot Autom 6:4967–4972. https://doi.org/10.1109/ICRA.2015.7139889

Zhou YM, Wagner D, Nuckols K et al (2019) Soft robotic glove with integrated sensing for intuitive grasping assistance post spinal cord injury. Proc IEEE Int Conf Robot Autom 5:9059–9065. https://doi.org/10.1109/ICRA.2019.8794367

Chapter 4
A Multi-segment Mechanism-Based Hand Exoskeleton: Motion Planning and Finger Structure Optimization

This chapter presents the development, modeling, and analysis of a multi-segment mechanism for a hand rehabilitation exoskeleton driven by a single layer of steel spring, capable of assisting both the extension and flexion of the fingers in alignment with natural human finger motion patterns. The multi-segment mechanism's inherent simplicity and flexibility enhance the device's overall performance, while its compliance ensures safety for human-robotic interaction. Furthermore, a tau-jerk motion planning approach, coupled with an exoskeleton finger structure optimization method, has been incorporated into the design and control system to ensure the exoskeleton's finger movements closely mirror human finger motions. Experimental results demonstrate that the hand motions generated by the exoskeleton, using our proposed tau-jerk motion planning method, exhibit superior conformity to human finger motions compared to commonly used methods, such as cubic polynomial interpolation and 3-4-5 polynomial interpolation for hand rehabilitation exoskeleton design.

4.1 Introduction

Bidirectional support, involving both finger extension and flexion, is crucial for effective hand rehabilitation (Iqbal et al. 2014). However, a wide range of existing devices such as those described in the literatures (Connelly et al. 2010; Yap et al. 2015a, 2015b; Polygerinos et al. 2013, 2015) as well as the one we described in Chap. 3 only provide finger flexion assistance. To enable bidirectional motion transmission, Borboni et al. (2016) introduced a hand exoskeleton powered by tendon-like cables in which the tendon serves as a tension element to assist finger extension, while during flexion, it behaves as a compressed flexible beam guided by linear rails mounted on the distal segments of the glove. Arata et al. (2013) developed an exoskeleton featuring a three-layer sliding spring mechanism to enable smooth and adaptive

M. Li and B. He, *Intention-Controlled Hand Rehabilitation for Stroke Survivors*,
https://doi.org/10.1007/978-981-95-4196-6_4

motion. The serially connected compliant elements are the most interesting feature of this hand exoskeleton mechanism. It has a potential to provide both safe human–robot interaction and biomechanically correct finger motions.

Motor recovery is shown to be greatly influenced by sensorimotor experience after stroke (Heo et al. 2012), ideally maintaining normal movements during rehabilitation training (Reinkensmeyer et al. 2004). To interpret human motor control and trajectory planning from the perspective of neuroscience and cognitive science, many internal model concepts have been proposed (Flash et al. 2013). However, currently, the motion patterns and strategies of fingers have not been fully considered in the design and control of hand exoskeletons (Vaz et al. 2017).

Due to the adaptability and intricate structure of the human hand, challenges still exist in designing hand exoskeleton robots for motor rehabilitation purposes with all the desired features such as simplicity, flexibility, safe human-robotic interaction, bi-directional actuation capability, affordability, portability, and conformity to human motion patterns. In this chapter, we present an overview of the design, modelling, and analysis of a mechanism with multiple segments actuated by a single layer of steel spring, capable of providing assistance for both finger extension and flexion. The steel spring can be manually slid forth and back, enabling the transmission of force in both directions while allowing for the development of a compact and cost-effective mechanism. Owing to the intrinsic characteristics of this multi-segment mechanism, the flexibility and simplicity of the device have been enhanced. Its flexibility ensures safe human-exoskeleton interface. Moreover, a tau-jerk motion planning and exoskeleton finger structure optimization method are proposed to make the exoskeleton finger motions in accordance with the motion patterns of the human fingers. Being conformity to human motion patterns and safe human–robot interaction are the key features of this hand exoskeleton.

The following sections detail the multi-segment mechanism design, kinematic modeling, motion planning, and optimization methods. We then present the experimental evaluation process and results, concluding with insights drawn from the validation studies.

4.2 Design Overview

The target users for the hand exoskeleton are stroke patients at the flaccid paralysis stage, who are incapable of opening or closing their hands. The primary clinical manifestations of this stage include muscle weakness, loss of active motor ability, and the disappearance of voluntary motor control (Kamper et al. 2006). At this stage, passive training is the primary rehabilitation method for improving hand functionality. The exoskeleton is designed with minimal interference with daily activities and is capable of generating sufficient forces for finger flexion and extension. The range of motion should ideally mirror that of a natural finger, or be slightly reduced to avoid causing strain or discomfort.

Our exoskeleton is intended for Continuous Passive Motion (CPM) rehabilitation training. CPM involves the passive movement of a patient's joint, either by a physiotherapist or by a rehabilitation robot, following a predefined motion sequence over a set period. During this process, external forces acting on the patient's joints should not exceed physiological values and must respect the degrees-of-freedom (DOF) of the joints (Borboni et al. 2016). Research has shown that CPM is an effective rehabilitation therapy for neurological patients (Hu et al. 2009; Giudice 1990; Seitz and Dinse 2007; Winter et al. 2011). It should be noted that CPM does not require high precision in monitoring finger movements (Borboni et al. 2016).

Based on these considerations, we propose a rigid-flexible integrated robot configuration for the hand exoskeleton, initially presented in our previous publication (Zhu et al. 2018). In this design, each finger is driven by a single actuator for both flexion and extension, ensuring a compact and efficient device. A multi-segment structure incorporating a spring layer is used to enhance adaptability and prevent joint misalignment issues during motion. As shown in Fig. 4.1, the spring layer bends and slides according to the linear motion input from the actuator. When attached to the finger, the structure supports the flexion and extension motion of the finger. The finger actuator exhibits greater bending at the joints compared to the finger segments, which led to a design where the sections above the joints are made thinner than those located at the distal, proximal, and metacarpal phalanges. This design ensures minimal daily activity interference. The device's width is limited to 20 mm to ensure a comfortable fit on the dorsal side of the finger, while also matching the natural width of the finger.

4.3 Kinematic Model

In this multi-segment mechanism, there are many parameters that can affect the bending profile. In order to simplify the kinematic model, we assume that the flexible strip at the segments between finger joints maintains a flat state during the entire process and the flexible strip at the joints segments bends circular-arc-shaped with a constant curvature at a certain instant (see Fig. 4.1b). The motor travel can be presented as

$$\begin{aligned} S &= S_1 + S_2 + S_3 \\ &= \frac{1}{2}\left(\frac{l_1}{\tan\frac{\theta_1}{2}}\theta_1 + \frac{l_2}{\tan\frac{\theta_2}{2}}\theta_2 + \frac{l_3}{\tan\frac{\theta_3}{2}}\theta_3\right) + h(\theta_1+\theta_2+\theta_3) \\ &\quad - (l_1+l_2+l_3) \end{aligned} \tag{4.1}$$

where l_1, l_2, l_3, d_1, d_2, and d_3, are the segment lengths; h is the distance between the flexible strip and the Velcro; θ_1, θ_2, and θ_3 are the joint angles of MCP, PIP, and DIP (see Fig. 4.1c). For a single joint, if h is fixed, the required motor travel to reach

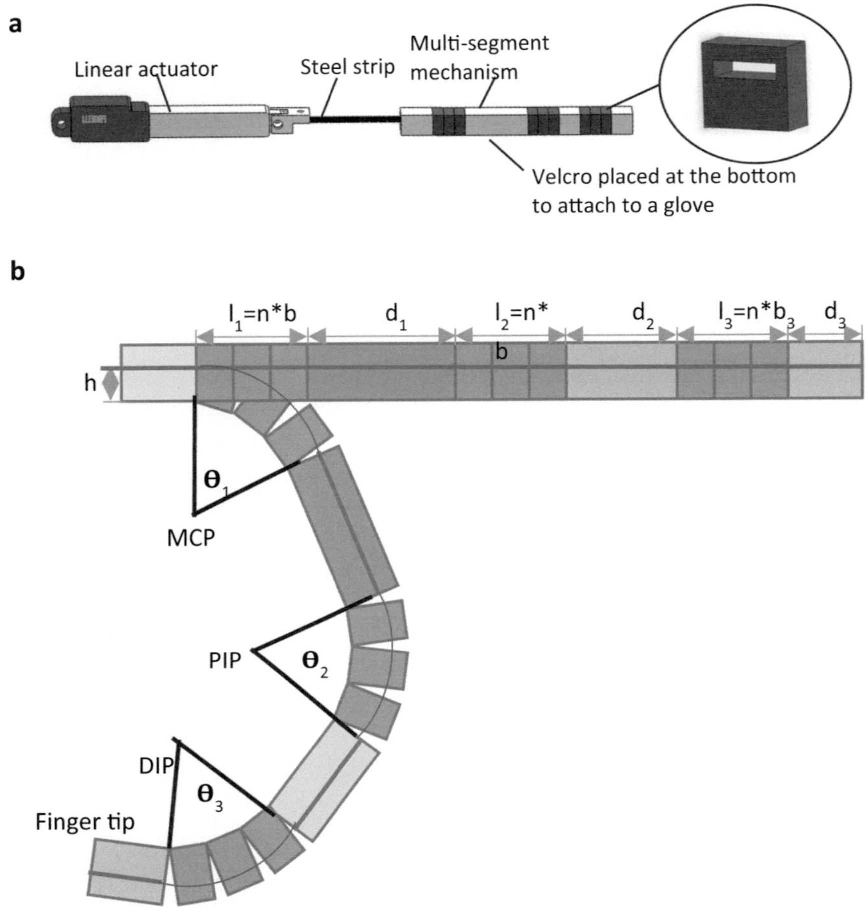

Fig. 4.1 Design of the finger exoskeleton: **a** overview of the exoskeleton actuator, **b** the multi-segment mechanism design showing the segment lengths, joint angles, the distance between the flexible strip and the Velcro

certain joint angle is getting smaller when l becomes larger. If l is fixed, the required motor travel to reach certain joint angle is getting smaller when h is smaller.

In order to validate this kinematic model, the multi-segment mechanism was modelled using three-dimensional finite element modeling (FEM), as shown in Fig. 4.2. The material properties of the segments, the strip, and the Velcro used in this FE model are shown in Table 4.1.

There was difference between the simulation result and the kinematic model for each finger. A correction factor μ was added to the kinematic model of each finger (see Eq. 4.2). The correction factors were 0.62, 0.58, 0.56, 0.58, and 0.59 for thumb, index, middle, ring, and little fingers.

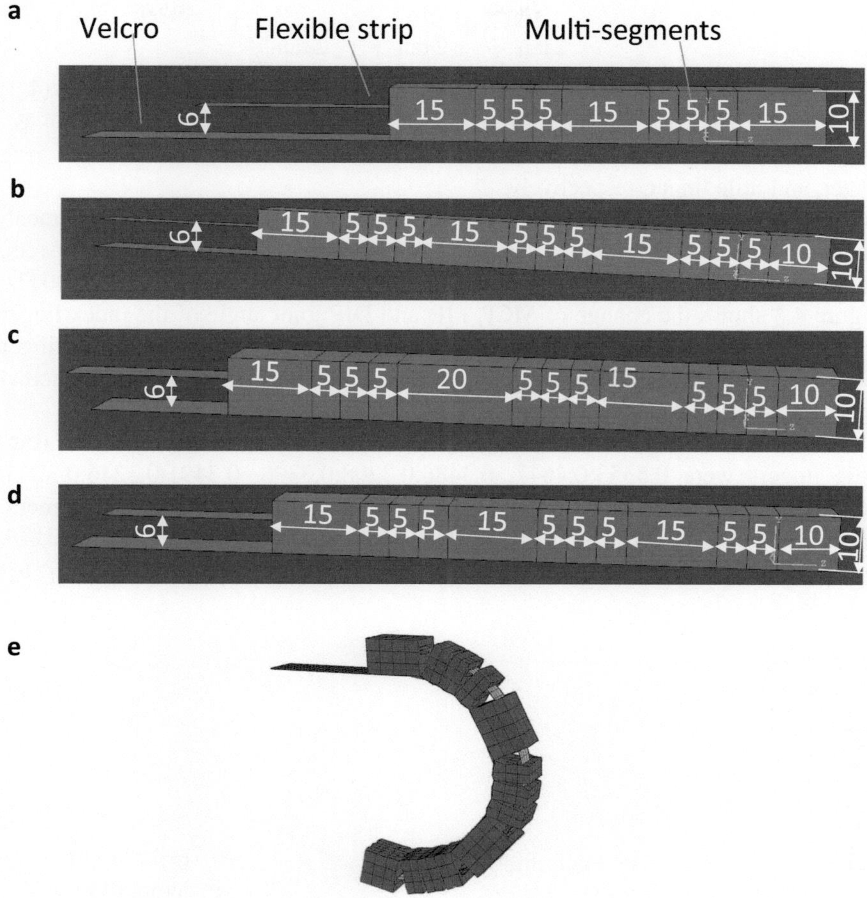

Fig. 4.2 3D modelling of the bending behavior of the multi-segment mechanism: **a** thumb, **b** index finger and ring finger, **c** middle finger, **d** little finger, and **e** an example of bending result

Table 4.1 Material parameters incorporated into the finite element model

	Mass density (kg/m^3)	Young's modulus (Pa)	Poisson's ratio
Segments	1200	1.0×10^9	0.25
Flexible strip	7900	2.5×10^9	0.3
Velcro	1540	28,300	0.4

$$S = \mu_i[(\frac{l_{i1}}{2\tan\frac{\theta_{i1}}{2}} + \frac{l_{i2}}{2\tan\frac{\theta_{i2}}{2}} + \frac{l_{i3}}{2\tan\frac{\theta_{i3}}{2}}) + h(\theta_{i1} + \theta_{i2} + \theta_{i3}) - (l_{i1} + l_{i2} + l_{i3})] \tag{4.2}$$

where i = 1, 2, 3, 4, 5 correspond to the thumb, index finger, middle finger, ring finger, and little finger, respectively.

An experiment was conducted to validate the simulation. During the experiment, finger movements were captured using a VICON system. The motion capture system, comprising ten T40 MX cameras, recorded movements at a sampling rate of 500 Hz. Figure 4.3 shows the change of MCP, PIP, and DIP joint angle of the index finger with linear motor stroke. The average errors for MCP, PIP, and DIP of index finger were 3.77, 0.68, and 3.22%. We consider that the simulation results fit the actual situations well.

For the simulation, the ratios of θ_1: θ_2: θ_3 of thumb, index, middle, ring, little fingers were 0.5353:0.4647, 0.3486:0.3208:0.3306, 0.3491:0.3246:0.3263, 0.3486:0.3208:0.3306, and 0.3741:0.3662:0.2598 respectively. For the experiment, the ratios were 0.5311: 0.4689, 0.3291: 0.3468: 0.3241, 0.3373:0.3519:0.3108, 0.3321: 0.3564: 0.3115, 0.3728: 0.3571: 0.2701 respectively. The ratios of θ_1: θ_2:

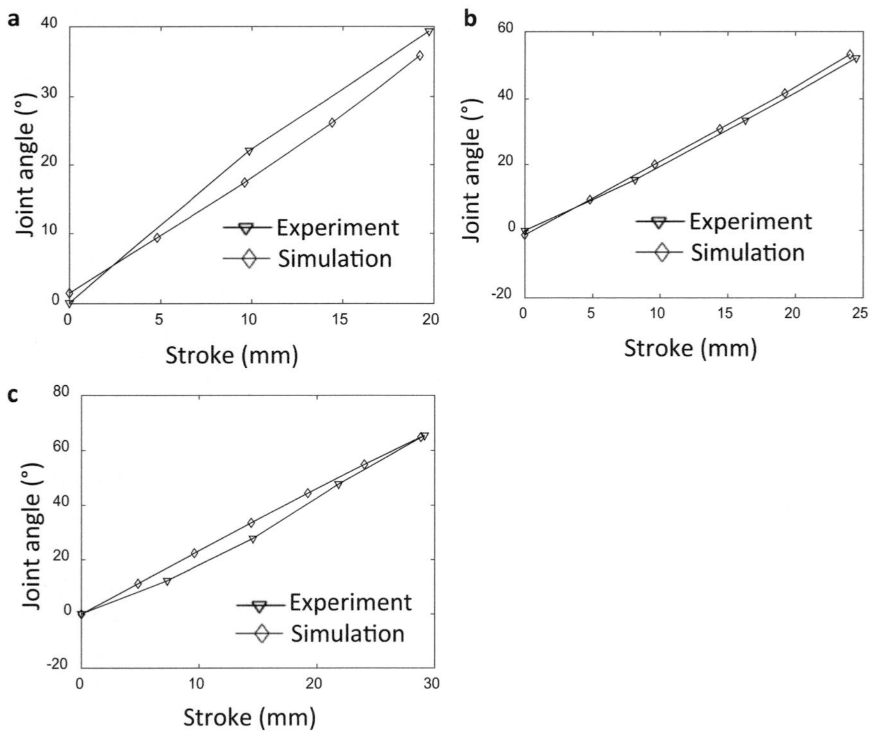

Fig. 4.3 Experimental results and simulation results: **a** MCP, **b** PIP, and **c** DIP

θ_3 of fingers were similar to the ratios of l_1:l_2:l_3. Considering the angle ratios, the finger model was formulated as the following (see Eq. 4.3).

$$\begin{cases} \mu_i[(\frac{l_{i1}}{2\tan\frac{\theta_{i1}}{2}} + h)\theta_{i1} - l_{i1}] = \frac{l_{i1}}{l_{i1}+l_{i2}+l_{i3}} S \\ \theta_{i2} = \frac{l_{i2}}{l_{i1}}\theta_{i1} \\ \theta_{i3} = \frac{l_{i3}}{l_{i1}}\theta_{i1} \end{cases} \quad (4.3)$$

4.4 Tau-Jerk Motion Planning

Motor recovery is greatly influenced by sensorimotor experience after stroke (Heo et al. 2012), ideally maintaining normal movements during rehabilitation training (Reinkensmeyer et al. 2004). Movements of the hand rehabilitation robot should be in conformity to human hand motion patterns. This ensures that patients experience the hand motions of healthy humans. Various studies have highlighted the importance of understanding human motion strategies to enhance the interaction between robots and human users (Loureiro et al. 2003). Hand closing-opening exercise is often used in hand rehabilitation. Cubic polynomial interpolation and 3-4-5 polynomial interpolation are often used in motion planning for hand rehabilitation robots. In contrast, general tau theory—developed by cognitive science researchers—provides a model that describes natural motion patterns as animals (including humans) approach a target position (Regan and Gray 2009; Delafield-Butt et al. 2012; Lee 2004). In this work, we introduce a tau-jerk motion planning method for hand rehabilitation robot design and control, a method first presented in our previous publication (Li et al. 2019), which we further validate through additional experiments.

In general tau theory, time-to-contact and time-to-collision, which refers to the remaining time of a moment before contact and collision, respectively, during target approaching or catching, have become important clues for researchers in cognitive science to reveal the motion patterns of animals approaching and catching a target object (Regan and Gray 2009; Lee 1998). All purposeful movements entail managing the closure of action gaps, namely, the separations between the current states animals are in and the goal states to be achieved by actions. Tau τ serves as an indicator of an action-gap and is considered the sole measure utilized by humans or animals to regulate the closing of such a gap. Here we define tau τ as.

$$\tau(t) = \frac{\theta(t)}{\dot{\theta}(t)}, \quad (4.4)$$

where $\theta(t)$ is the angular error of the joint at time t; $\dot{\theta}(t)$ is the angular velocity at the moment t of the joint.

Here we propose to use a jerk-guided tau strategy for finger motion planning. $\theta(t)$ is assumed to be closed with a constant *jerk* value (the first derivative of acceleration).

We assume that such movements are inherently guided by tau-coupling the action-gap, $\theta(t)$, to an internally generated reference action-gap, j(t), through adherence to the τ_j-guidance equation.

$$\tau_\theta(t) = k \cdot \tau_j(t), \tag{4.5}$$

where k, which defines the kinematic characteristics of the movement, such as the patterns of velocity and acceleration profiles, is constant during a movement and is presumed to be established by the brain. $\tau_j(t)$ is the internally generated reference action-gap; $\tau_\theta(t)$ is the action-gap of joint angle.

The kinematic parameters of this motion can be calculated as

$$\begin{cases} \theta(t) = \theta - \frac{\theta}{T^{\frac{3}{k}}}(T^3 - t^3)^{\frac{1}{k}} \\ \dot{\theta}(t) = \frac{3\theta t^2}{k_A T^{\frac{3}{k}}}(T_j^3 - t^3)^{\frac{1-k}{k}} \\ \ddot{\theta}(t) = \frac{-3\theta t}{kT^{\frac{3}{k}}}(\frac{3-k}{k} - 2T^3)(T^3 - t^3)^{\frac{1-2k}{k}} \end{cases} \tag{4.6}$$

where θ is the joint angle; k is a coupling factor that determines the trajectory; T is motion duration. When and only when $0 < k < 0.5$, the closing velocity and acceleration are all zero, which means the motion is smooth and steady.

4.5 Optimized Trajectory and Exoskeleton Finger Structure

The hand rehabilitation robot design should allow some customization to hand size, different desired bending profiles, different patient statuses, and different stages of rehabilitation. A standard customization process should be established. The process of personalized customization is shown in this section.

The work of the motor did during the time of $T_{\rm j}$ is $W = \int_0^{T_j} fSdt$. For a given structure of the multi-segment mechanism, joint angle, and movement time, an optimized k (a coupling factor that determines the trajectory) with minimum motor work can be acquired. We assume the structure of the multi-segment mechanism should be as small as possible. Here we introduce another parameter, namely structural area S.

$$\mathrm{S} = \mathrm{lh} \tag{4.7}$$

The work and structural area are normalized to remove the dimension.

$$\begin{cases} W_{nor} = \frac{W - W_{\min}}{W_{\max} - W_{\min}} \\ S_{nor} = \frac{s - s_{\min}}{s_{\max} - s_{\min}} \end{cases} \tag{4.8}$$

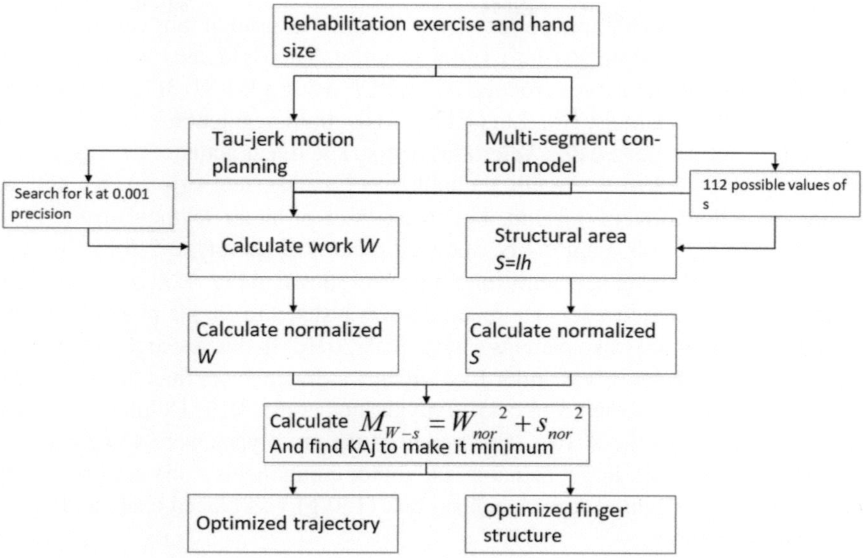

Fig. 4.4 The process of rehabilitation exoskeleton finger design and trajectory design for specific rehabilitation exercise and hand size

We define M_{W-s} to combine these two parameters:

$$M_{W-s} = W_{nor}^2 + s_{nor}^2 \tag{4.9}$$

As shown in Fig. 4.4, the desired rehabilitation exercise is first determined. The information of joint angles and movement duration of this exercise movement is then acquired. Two principles, minimum work and minimum structural area, are used to search for the optimized coupling factor K_{Aj}, which determines the bending profile, bending trajectory, and the optimized finger structure.

4.6 Evaluation Experiments

An experiment was conducted to verify the proposed rehabilitation exoskeleton design and motion planning method. Two 24-year-old healthy male subjects with a small hand and a larger hand participated in this experiment. The desired motions were from hand open to a gesture shown in Fig. 4.5. The time duration of motion is 4s. Using the proposed finger trajectory and exoskeleton finger structure optimization method, the optimized structures and trajectories were acquired for the specific hand motions and the hand sizes (see Table 4.2). Two prototypes of the hand exoskeletons were then developed. Figure 4.6a shows a picture of the prototype 1 for subject 1.

A 3D Systems MJP3600 rapid prototyping machine was used to fabricate the mechanism's components from VisiJet Crystal material. The rigid section, designed to mount the linear actuator, was produced from PLA using a D3020 3D printer (Shenzhen Sundystar Technology Co., Ltd., China). The multi-segment mechanisms were secured to a textile glove using Velcro fasteners. The linear actuators we used here are L12-50–210-12-I from Firgelli Technologies Ca. The steel strip has a length of 80 mm and a thickness of 0.3 mm. The thicknesses of finger segments (unit: mm) are shown in Fig. 4.6b. Figure 4.6c shows a picture of prototype 2 for subject 2. The thicknesses of finger segments (unit: mm) are shown in Fig. 4.6d. A lightweight design is a critical requirement for rehabilitation systems to enable practical use by a broad population of stroke patients (Nycz et al. 2016). In our research, the desired weight of the exoskeleton was under 1 kg which was much lower than that of current existing hand exoskeletons (3 to 5 kg (Polygerinos et al. 2015; Delph et al. 2013; CyberGlove Systems Inc 2016)). The weight of the prototypes were 435 g and 443 g comprising the glove, finger actuator, and motor components - this is significantly below the target weight (1 kg). A control box (150 g) was placed aside adding no extra load to the arm.

In order to evaluate the proposed motion planning and exoskeleton finger structure optimization method, we compared the subject's hand performing the motion

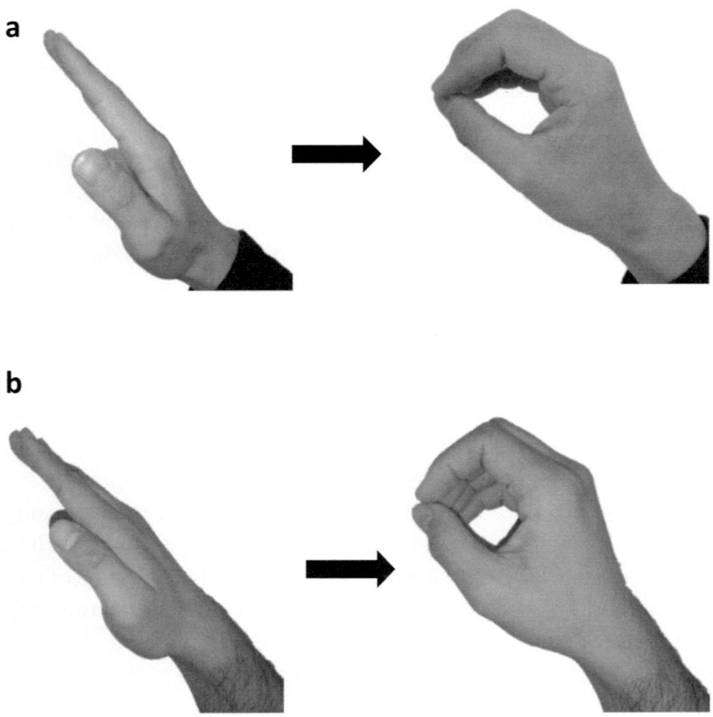

Fig. 4.5 The desired hand motions for **a** subject 1 and **b** subject 2

Table 4.2 Structural parameters (l × h in mm) and Tau factors

Subject	Finger	MCP structural parameters (l × h, in mm)	MCP tau factor	PIP structural parameters (l × h, in mm)	PIP tau factor	DIP structural parameters (l × h, in mm)	DIP tau factor
Subject1	Thumb	6 × 6	0.4656	7 × 6	0.4352	Null	Null
	Index	6 × 6	0.4656	9 × 6	0.3733	7 × 6	0.4352
	Middle	6 × 6	0.4656	10 × 6	0.3429	7 × 6	0.4352
	Ring	7 × 6	0.4352	10 × 6	0.3429	6 × 6	0.4656
	Little	6 × 6	0.4656	10 × 6	0.3429	7 × 6	0.4352
Subject2	Thumb	6 × 6	0.4656	7 × 6	0.4352	Null	Null
	Index	6 × 6	0.4656	9 × 6	0.3733	7 × 6	0.4352
	Middle	6 × 6	0.4656	10 × 6	0.3429	7 × 6	0.4352
	Ring	7 × 6	0.4352	10 × 6	0.3429	6 × 6	0.4656
	Little	6 × 6	0.4656	10 × 6	0.3429	7 × 6	0.4352

actively, motion planned by cubic polynomial interpolation, 3-4-5 polynomial interpolation, and the proposed method, as well as the motion of the subject's hand assisted by the exoskeleton. While the process was ongoing, finger movements were recorded using the VICON system. Twenty-one reflective dome-shaped markers, each with a diameter of 9 mm, were affixed to the finger joints of the participants. The procedure was replicated three times under identical conditions. The research involving human participants was examined and authorized by the Institutional Review Board of Xi'an Jiaotong University.

Joint angle relative standard error was calculated using the following Eq. (4.10)

$$e_{\theta_i} = \frac{\sqrt{\frac{1}{n}[e_{\theta_i(t)}]^2}}{q} \times 100\% \tag{4.10}$$

where $e_{\theta_i(t)}$ is the absolute error between the actual joint angle and the desired joint angle of joint i at moment t; q is the joint angle change from the beginning to the end of the motion; n is the sample number.

Fingertip trajectory relative standard error was calculated using Eq. (4.11)

$$e_{tr_i} = \frac{\sqrt{\frac{1}{n}\{[e_{x_i(t)}]^2 + [e_{y_i(t)}]^2\}}}{D} \times 100\% \tag{4.11}$$

where $e_{x_i(t)}$ isthe absolute difference between the measured and target fingertip trajectories at moment t along axis x; $e_{y_i(t)}$ is the absolute error between the actual fingertip trajectory and the desired trajectory of finger i at moment t along axis y; D is the fingertip displacement from the beginning to the end of the motion; n is the sample number.

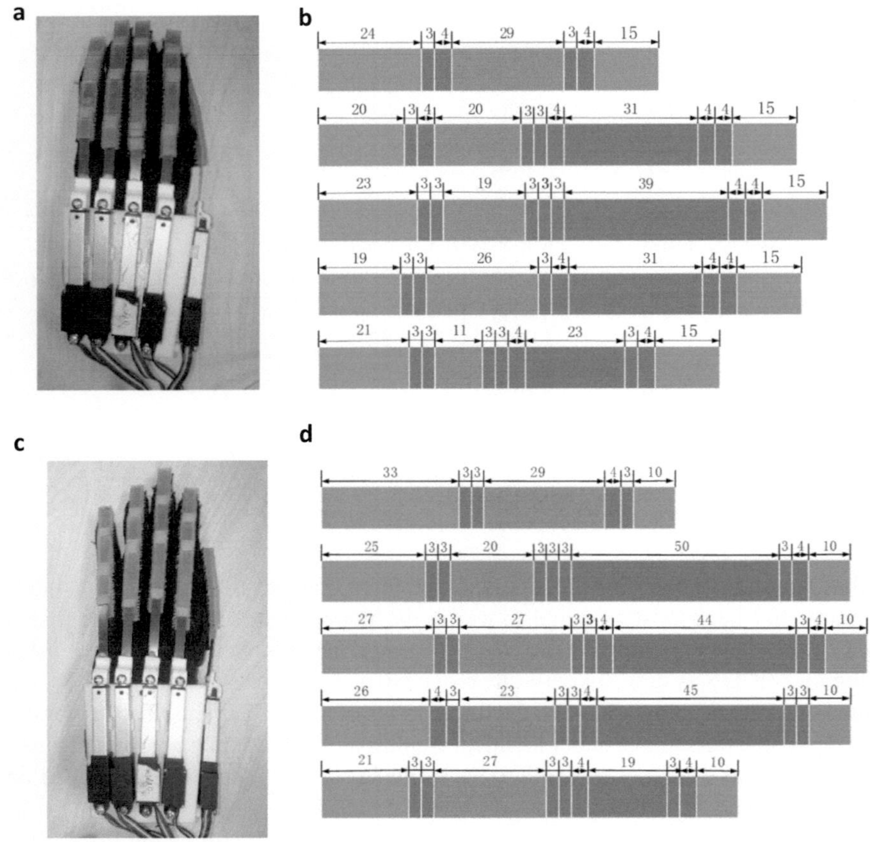

Fig. 4.6 The hand exoskeletons prototypes and dimensions of thumb, index/ring finger, middle finger, and little finger for subject 1 (shown in **a** and **b**) and subject 2 (shown in **c** and **d**)

4.7 Experimental Results

Three types of hand motion results, including (1) finger motion planning results using cubic polynomial interpolation, (2) finger motion planning results using 3–4-5 polynomial interpolation, and (3) the hand motion results driven by the exoskeletons, were compared to the subjects' bare hand motions. Figures 4.7 and 4.8 show the index finger motions of subject 1 and 2. Figures 4.9 and 4.10 show the thumb motions of subject 1 and 2. Table 4.3 shows the average joint angle errors (relative standard errors and absolute errors) and fingertip trajectory errors of each subject. Figure 4.11a shows the joint angle errors of the hand motions compared to the subjects' bare hand motions. A student t-test was used to verify the significance of the joint angle error differences between the motion planning results and the subjects' bare hand motions. The sample size was 84 (14 joints $\times$ 3 trials $\times$ 2 subjects). The hand motion results driven by the exoskeletons had significantly lower joint angle relative standard errors compared to motion planning results using cubic polynomial interpolation ($p = 9.71 \times 10^{-25}$) and 3-4-5 polynomial interpolation ($p = 2.57 \times 10^{-31}$).

Figure 4.11b shows the fingertip trajectory errors of the planned motions using cubic polynomial interpolation, 3-4-5 polynomial interpolation, and the hand motion results driven by the exoskeletons compared to the target hand motion. A student t-test was used to verify the significance of the fingertip trajectory error differences between the motion planning results and the subjects' bare hand motions. The sample size was 30 (5 fingers × 3 trials × 2 subjects). The hand motion results driven by the exoskeletons had significantly lower relative standard errors of trajectory compared to motion planning results using cubic polynomial interpolation ($p = 4.37 \times 10^{-20}$) and 3-4-5 polynomial interpolation ($p = 1.45 \times 10^{-21}$).

In general, the subjects' hand motions driven by the exoskeleton fitted very well to the desired motions with an average joint angle error of 7.46% (1.16°) and fingertip

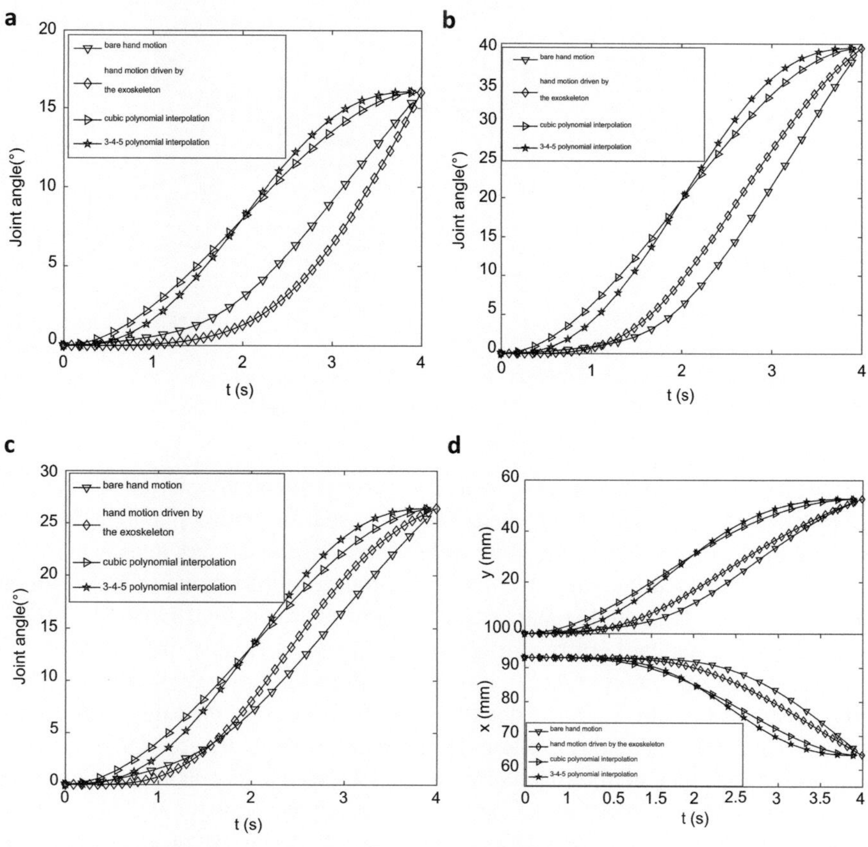

Fig. 4.7 Comparison of different motion planning results and the actual motion of the exoskeleton index finger of subject 1: **a** MCP, **b** PIP, **c** DIP, and **d** fingertip trajectory

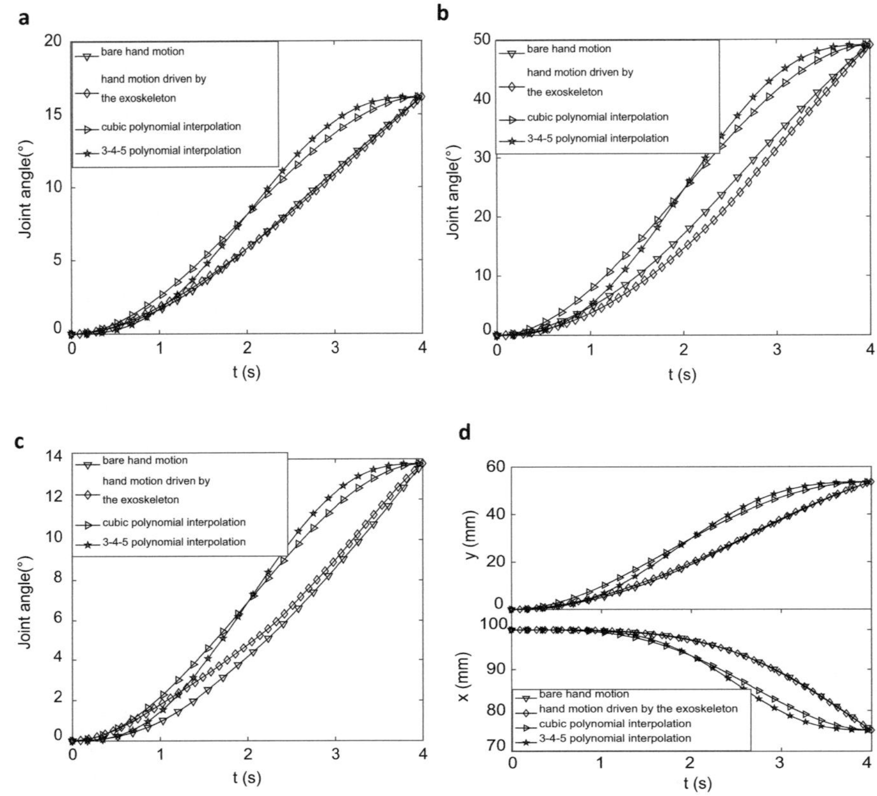

Fig. 4.8 Comparison of different motion planning results and the actual motion of the exoskeleton index finger of subject 2: **a** MCP, **b** PIP, **c** DIP, and **d** fingertip trajectory

trajectory of 2.21% (0.71 mm). Compared to cubic polynomial interpolation and 3-4-5 polynomial interpolation that are commonly used for motion planning for hand rehabilitation exoskeleton design, the exoskeleton using the tau-jerk motion planning method we proposed had significantly better conformity to human finger motion patterns (average joint angle relative standard error: 7.46 versus 15.70 and 17.09%, average relative standard errors of trajectory: 2.21 versus 16.39% and 17.71%).

The steel spring incorporated in our design allows the exoskeleton to integrate the advantages of both rigid and flexible systems. It delivers the high force output typical of rigid exoskeletons while enabling natural finger flexion and extension, which simplifies the overall finger structure and reduces mechanical complexity. In comparison to the exoskeleton developed by Arata et al. (Arata et al. 2013), which utilizes a mechanism with three layers of springs, the design we proposed incorporates a reduced number of sliding springs, resulting in a more compact and efficient system. Additionally, unlike the exoskeleton proposed by Borboni et al. (Borboni

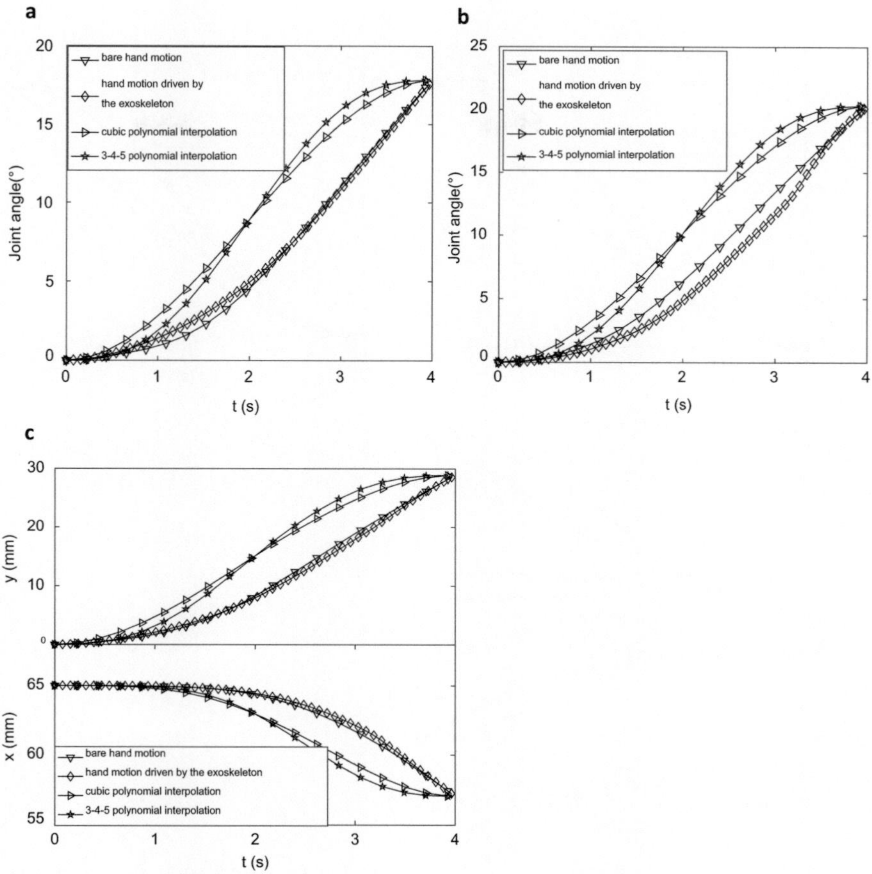

Fig. 4.9 Comparison of different motion planning results and the actual motion of the exoskeleton thumb of subject 1: **a** CP, **b** IP, and **d** fingertip trajectory

et al. 2016), which requires a separate portable trolley to carry air compressor, pneumatic components, and electronics, our design eliminates these extra components, making the entire device significantly smaller and more portable.

We also introduced a tau-jerk motion planning and exoskeleton finger structure optimization method, ensuring that the exoskeleton's finger motions closely align with human hand motion patterns. Evaluation experiments demonstrated that our tau-jerk motion planning method resulted in better conformity to natural finger motion patterns compared to conventional cubic polynomial interpolation and 3-4-5 polynomial interpolation, which are commonly used in hand rehabilitation exoskeleton design. Specifically, the desired motion and the actual hand motion driven by the exoskeleton matched very well, with an average joint angle error of less than 1.5° and an average fingertip trajectory error of less than 1 mm.

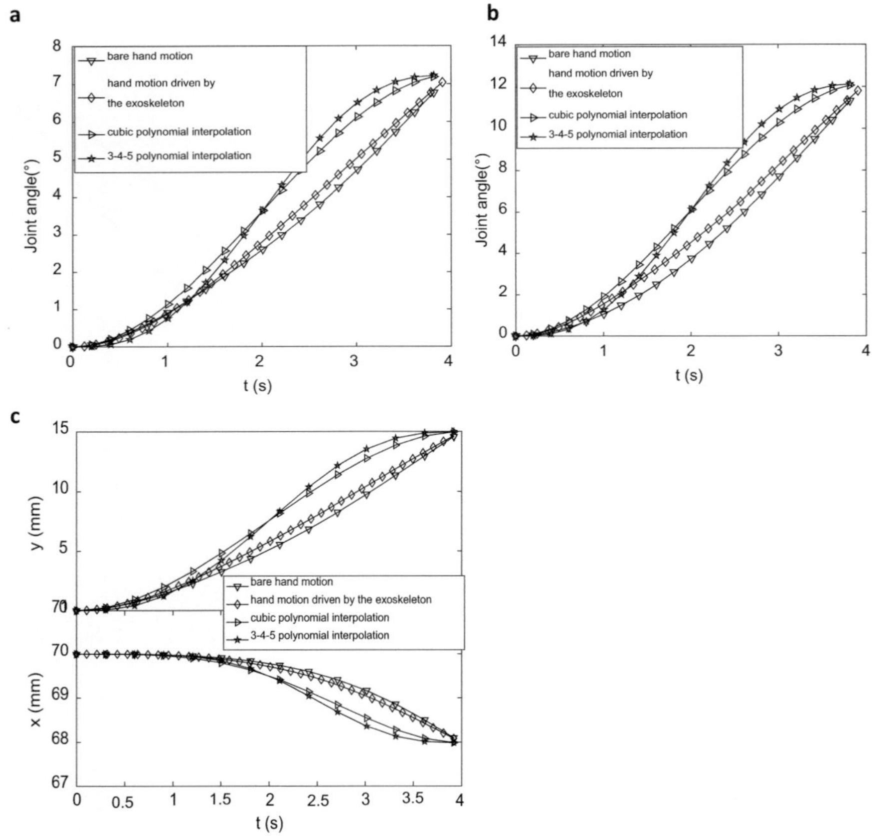

Fig. 4.10 Comparison of different motion planning results and the actual motion of the exoskeleton thumb of subject 2: **a** CP, **b** IP, and **d** fingertip trajectory

4.8 Two-DOF Finger Exoskeleton

This design can avoid the problem that the rotation centers of the robot and the human hand do not overlap caused by rigid exoskeletons, and can also avoid the problems of nonlinear deformation and difficult control existing in flexible exoskeletons. However, each finger is driven by an electric push rod, which makes the movement of other skeletal fingers relatively slow, with fewer degrees of freedom and smaller output force. Meanwhile, since the material used for exoskeletons is photosensitive resin, its strength is insufficient and fatigue fracture often occurs during use.

Providing multiple DOFs for each finger can greatly enhance gripping flexibility and enhance the joint's functionality. To further this, we proposed a hand exoskeleton featuring a similar multi-segment mechanism, driven by two motors, offering two DOFs per finger (Shi et al. 2023). This configuration enables the exoskeleton to achieve a larger range of motion (MCP 85°, PIP 65°, and DIP 67°). The gripping

Table 4.3 The average joint angle errors and fingertip trajectory errors

Subject	Motion type	Joint angle RSE (%)	Joint angle absolute errors (°)	Trajectory RSE (%)	Trajectory absolute errors (mm)
Subject 1	Hand motion driven by the exoskeleton	7.13	1.23	2.39	0.82
	Motion planning using cubic polynomial interpolation	16.59	3.49	17.56	8.21
	Motion planning using 3-4-5 polynomial interpolation	17.78	3.50	18.67	8.15
Subject 2	Hand motion driven by the exoskeleton	7.79	1.23	2.02	0.60
	Motion planning using cubic polynomial interpolation	14.81	3.00	15.21	6.59
	Motion planning using 3-4-5 polynomial interpolation	16.40	3.00	16.74	6.65

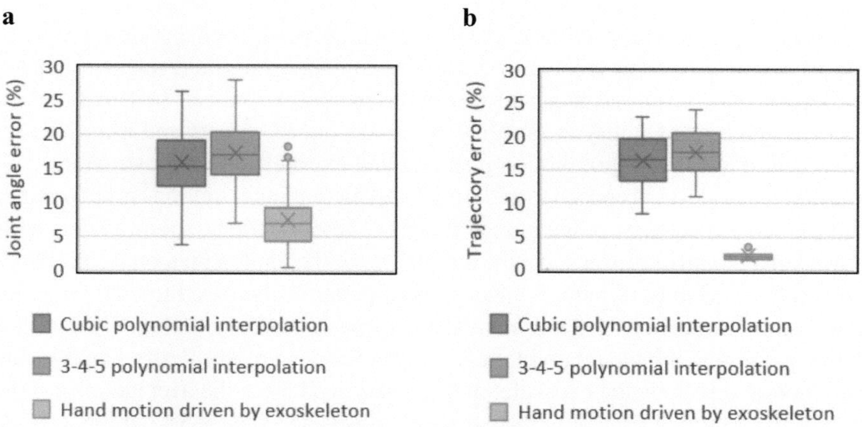

Fig. 4.11 **a** The joint angle errors and **b** the fingertip trajectory errors of the planned motions using cubic polynomial interpolation, 3-4-5 polynomial interpolation, and the hand motion results driven by the exoskeletons compared to the target hand motion

capability was quantitatively assessed, showing an average fingertip force of 3.59 N, with the exoskeleton capable of independently holding a weight of approximately 1 kg and gripping a 40 mm diameter cylinder with a maximum weight of 550 g. Due to the larger driven units compared to those used in the exoskeleton described in this chapter, it is difficult to include five fingers in this design. Therefore, at the

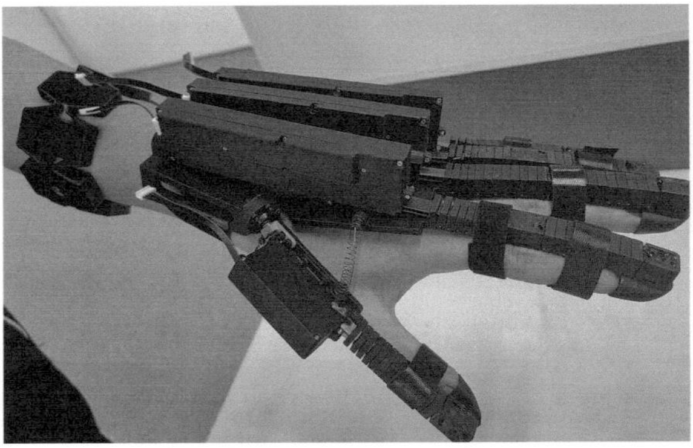

Fig. 4.12 A five-finger hand exoskeleton with two DOFs each finger

beginning this design supports only three fingers. Later, we managed to make a hand exoskeleton with five fingers by combining the actuation of the middle finger and ring finger (see Fig. 4.12).

4.9 Conclusion

In this chapter, we proposed an exoskeleton with a multi-segment structure actuated by a single layer of steel spring, capable of supporting both finger extension and flexion. The proposed mechanism has the flexibility that can be beneficial for achieving high adaptability in grasping complex-shaped objects and improve user safety. Moreover, a tau-jerk motion planning and exoskeleton finger structure optimization method was proposed to make the exoskeleton finger motions in accordance with the motion patterns of the human fingers. The evaluation experimental results showed that the exoskeleton using the tau-jerk motion planning method we proposed had better conformity to human finger motion patterns compared to cubic polynomial interpolation and 3-4-5 polynomial interpolation that are commonly used for motion planning for hand rehabilitation exoskeleton design. The desired motion and hand motion driven by the exoskeleton fitted very well since the average joint angle error of hand motion driven by the exoskeleton was less than 1.5° and the average fingertip trajectory error of hand motion generated by the exoskeleton was less than 1 mm. Features of our hand exoskeleton include: low complexity, compact design, bidirectional actuation, cost-effectiveness, and portability, in conformity to human motion patterns, and safe human-robotic interaction.

References

Arata J, Ohmoto K, Gassert R et al (2013) A new hand exoskeleton device for rehabilitation using a three-layered sliding spring mechanism. In: Procceding IEEE international conference robotics automatiom, pp 3902–3907. https://doi.org/10.1109/ICRA.2013.6631126

Borboni A, Mor M, Faglia R (2016) Gloreha—hand robotic rehabilitation: design, mechanical model, and experiments. J Dyn Syst Meas Control 138:111003. https://doi.org/10.1115/1.4033831

Connelly L, Jia Y, Toro ML et al (2010) A pneumatic glove and immersive virtual reality environment for hand rehabilitative training after stroke. IEEE Trans Neural Syst Rehabil Eng 18:551–559. https://doi.org/10.1109/TNSRE.2010.2047588

Delafield-Butt JT, Pepping GJ, McCaig CD, Lee DN (2012) Prospective guidance in a free-swimming cell. Biol Cybern 106:283–293. https://doi.org/10.1007/s00422-012-0495-5

Delph MA, Fischer SA, Gauthier PW et al (2013) A soft robotic exomusculature glove with integrated sEMG sensing for hand rehabilitation. In: IEEE international conference on rehabilitation robotics, pp 1–7

Flash T, Meirovitch Y, Barliya A (2013) Models of human movement: trajectory planning and inverse kinematics studies. Rob Auton Syst 61:330–339. https://doi.org/10.1016/j.robot.2012.09.020

Giudice ML (1990) Effects of continuous passive motion and elevation on hand edema. Am J Occup Ther 44:914–921

Heo P, Gu GM, Lee S et al (2012) Current hand exoskeleton technologies for rehabilitation and assistive engineering. Int J Precis Eng Manuf 13:807–824. https://doi.org/10.1007/s12541-012-0107-2

Hu XL, Tong KY, Song R et al (2009) A comparison between electromyography-driven robot and passive motion device on wrist rehabilitation for chronic stroke. Neurorehabil Neural Repair 23:837–846. https://doi.org/10.1177/1545968309338191

CyberGlove Systems Inc. Cybergrasp. http://www.cyberglovesystems.com/cybergrasp. Accessed 16 Dec 2016

Iqbal J, Khan H, Tsagarakis NG, Caldwell DG (2014) A novel exoskeleton robotic system for hand rehabilitation—conceptualization to prototyping. Biocybern Biomed Eng 34:79–89. https://doi.org/10.1016/j.bbe.2014.01.003

Kamper DG, Fischer HC, Cruz EG, Rymer WZ (2006) Weakness is the primary contributor to finger impairment in chronic stroke. Arch Phys Med Rehabil 87:1262–1269. https://doi.org/10.1016/j.apmr.2006.05.013

Lee DN (1998) Guiding movement by coupling Taus. Ecol Psychol 10:221–250

Lee DN (2004) Tau in action in development. In: Action, perception & cognition in learning and development, p 58

Li M, Chen J, He B et al (2019) Motion planning and structure optimization of a multi-segment mechanism-based hand rehabilitation exoskeleton. Hsi-An Chiao Tung Ta Hsueh/J Xi'an Jiaotong Univ 53. https://doi.org/10.7652/xjtuxb201910001

Loureiro RUI, Amirabdollahian F, Topping M, Driessen B (2003) Upper limb robot mediated stroke therapy—GENTLE/s approach. Auton Robots 15Loureiro:35–51. https://doi.org/10.1023/A:1024436732030

Nycz CJ, Butzer T, Lambercy O et al (2016) Design and characterization of a lightweight and fully portable remote actuation system for use with a hand exoskeleton. IEEE Robot Autom Lett 1:976–983. https://doi.org/10.1109/LRA.2016.2528296

Polygerinos P, Wang Z, Galloway KC et al (2015) Soft robotic glove for combined assistance and at-home rehabilitation. Rob Auton Syst 73:135–143. https://doi.org/10.1016/j.robot.2014.08.014

Polygerinos P, Lyne S, Wang Z et al (2013) Towards a soft pneumatic glove for hand rehabilitation. In: IEEE International conference on intelligent robots and systems, pp 1512–1517

Regan D, Gray R (2009) General tau theory: evolution to date. Perception 38:837–858. https://doi.org/10.1068/ldmk-lee

Reinkensmeyer DJ, Emken JL, Cramer SC (2004) Robotics, motor learning, and neurologic recovery. Ann Rev Biomed Eng 6:497–525. https://doi.org/10.1146/annurev.bioeng.6.040803.140223

Seitz AR, Dinse HR (2007) A common framework for perceptual learning. Curr Opin Neurobiol 17:148–153

Shi Z, Li M, He B et al (2023) A hand exoskeleton using a multi-segment mechanism with two degrees-of-freedom for each finger. In: 2023 20th international conference on ubiquitous robots, UR

Vaz DV, Silva PL, Mancini MC et al (2017) Towards an ecologically grounded functional practice in rehabilitation. Hum Mov Sci 52:117–132. https://doi.org/10.1016/j.humov.2017.01.010

Winter J, Hunter S, Sim J, Crome P (2011) Hands-on therapy interventions for upper limb motor dysfunction following stroke. Cochr Database Syst Rev CD006609. https://doi.org/10.1002/14651858.CD006609.pub2

Yap HK, Goh JCH, Yeow RCH (2015a) Design and charaterization of soft actuator for hand rehabilitation application. In: Proceedings of European conference of the international federation for medical and biological engineering, pp 367–370

Yap HK, Jeong HL, Nasrallah F et al (2015b) A soft exoskeleton for hand assistive and rehabilitation application using pneumatic actuators with variable stiffness. In: 2015 IEEE international conference on robotics and automation (ICRA). IEEE, pp 4967–4972

Zhu S, Li M, Xu G et al (2018) Finger exoskeleton for rehabilitation of finger extension and flexion by multi-segment mechanism. Hsi-An Chiao Tung Ta Hsueh/J Xi'an Jiaotong Univ 52:17–22+121. https://doi.org/10.7652/xjtuxb201806003

Chapter 5
Attention-Controlled Hand and Wrist Rehabilitation Assistance with Affordable EEG Sensors: Design, Implementation, and Preliminary Evaluation

Effective rehabilitation for hand and wrist motor impairments relies on active patient involvement in therapeutic exercises. This chapter introduces an integrated attention-controlled rehabilitation system for the hand and wrist, using a low-cost electroencephalography (EEG) sensor to engage patients' focus in training sessions. The system incorporates a flexible wrist exoskeleton designed to support wrist flexion/extension and radial/ulnar deviation, alongside a hand exoskeleton featuring a hybrid soft-rigid multi-segment structure for finger flexion and extension. By establishing a brain-controlled switch activated by a threshold attention level measured via EEG, both exoskeletons enable user-driven, active rehabilitation. The design and development of the brain-controlled switch allow the system to operate when patients maintain a predefined level of attentiveness, encouraging their active participation in each exercise. Visual guidance is also integrated to help users concentrate, leading to a 95% success rate in system actuation across various experiments. The hand exoskeleton employs a unique mechanism that efficiently translates a single linear input into the required rotational movements for finger joints, achieving sufficient motion range for rehabilitation purposes. Experiments demonstrated that using a general attention threshold performed as well as customized thresholds, simplifying the setup process for specific patient groups. This chapter details the overall design, system integration, and experimental results, providing insights into the potential for using affordable EEG sensors to create intuitive, brain-controlled rehabilitation devices for upper-limb recovery.

M. Li and B. He, *Intention-Controlled Hand Rehabilitation for Stroke Survivors*,
https://doi.org/10.1007/978-981-95-4196-6_5

5.1 Introduction

The ability to control and use hand and wrist functions is crucial for daily activities and maintaining a high quality of life (Squeri et al. 2013; Heo et al. 2012). Even partial loss of hand or wrist function, often caused by neurological impairments such as stroke, can severely impact an individual's independence and ability to perform activities of daily living (ADLs) (Takahashi et al. 2008). Hand rehabilitation focuses on improving finger and wrist strength, range of motion, and motor accuracy, often through repetitive task-based exercises (Takahashi et al. 2008; Wolf et al. 2015; Carmeli et al. 2011; Kutner et al. 2010; Ueki et al. 2008). Traditionally, these rehabilitation exercises have required close supervision by therapists, which is effective but costly and time-consuming (Johansson 2011). As a result, many patients are unable to access the extensive therapy sessions necessary for optimal recovery (Maciejasz et al. 2014). Robotic rehabilitation technologies have emerged as promising solutions to address these limitations, offering assistance with repetitive movements and providing quantitative assessments of patient progress, which are essential for tailored rehabilitation programs (Krebs et al. 2007).

As we presented in Chap. 1, brain-computer interfaces (BCIs) have been introduced to promote active patient engagement in rehabilitation exercises (Li et al. 2018; Jiang et al. 2014a, 2014b). Studies have shown that active engagement in rehabilitation, driven by the user's movement intentions, can significantly enhance neuroplasticity, improving motor function and recovery (Li et al. 2018; Teo and Chew 2014). Traditional BCIs, however, often rely on complex and costly EEG devices with multi-channel electrode caps and require conductive gels, making them more suitable for research than for practical clinical use. There is a pressing need for user-friendly, affordable BCI solutions that offer acceptable accuracy and reliability, making rehabilitation more accessible both in clinical and home settings (Li et al. 2018; Dokkum et al. 2015).

This chapter explores attention-controlled assistive hand and wrist rehabilitation using an affordable EEG-based brain-controlled switch, offering a practical and accessible solution to encourage active patient engagement. By using a low-cost, easy-to-wear EEG sensor, patients can control a hand and wrist exoskeleton to assist with flexion and extension movements. This approach builds on the integration of soft-rigid combined mechanisms in hand exoskeleton design and a flexible wrist exoskeleton, addressing both the versatility and functional complexity required for effective hand and wrist rehabilitation. Using attention-based thresholds as control inputs, this system enables patients to engage in active rehabilitation, responding to their attention levels and encouraging focused participation without the inconvenience of traditional EEG systems.

The design of these exoskeletons incorporates features essential for safe, efficient, and intuitive rehabilitation. The hand exoskeleton incorporates a hybrid soft-rigid multi-segment structure, offering both flexion and extension support through a single-input system. This design minimizes joint misalignment issues, enhancing comfort and safety during use, while remaining compact and portable for ease of use in diverse settings. The wrist exoskeleton, similarly, facilitates active training with a minimalistic approach, using an attention-based BCI method as a substitute for traditional motor imagery (MI)-based systems, reducing complexity and increasing accessibility.

This chapter's primary contributions are the development of an affordable, attention-controlled system for hand and wrist rehabilitation, the experimental validation of attention thresholds in assisting movements, and the demonstration of how visual guidance can support patient concentration during training. By integrating active attention control and intuitive visual feedback, this system provides an effective, patient-centered approach to rehabilitation that is accessible, low-cost, and capable of delivering safe and effective therapy both in clinical environments and at home.

The rest of this chapter is organized as follows: Sect. 5.2 provides an overview of the proposed method's design. Section 5.3 details the design of the hand and wrist exoskeletons. Section 5.4 introduces the brain-controlled switch developed for these exoskeletons. Section 5.5 outlines the experimental protocol and presents the corresponding results. Finally, Sect. 5.6 offers a discussion of the findings and their implications.

5.2 Overall Design of the Proposed Brain-Controlled Hand and Wrist Rehabilitation

The brain-controlled hand and wrist rehabilitation system leverages attention-based control to enable active engagement in motor training through a combination of visual guidance and exoskeleton assistance, as illustrated in Fig. 5.1. This concept was presented in our previous studies (Li et al. 2019a, 2019b). Here, we reframe this concept. This system supports extension, flexion, radial deviation, and ulnar deviation movements of wrist, as well as finger flexion and extension for hand rehabilitation purposes. Both the hand and wrist rehabilitation devices are designed to be activated by the user's focus level, which is captured using an affordable EEG sensor and serves as a substitute for more traditional motor imagery-based control.

Incorporating insights from neuroscience, this system relies on the activation of mirror neurons to facilitate motor recovery. Mirror neurons are known to activate when an individual performs a movement, imagines a movement, or observes the movement performed by others, including robotic systems and virtual simulations (Oztop et al. 2013). This activation bridges the cognitive processes of vision and motion, which is highly beneficial for motor recovery. To engage these mirror neurons, the system displays a motion demonstration on a screen, serving as a form of visual guidance. This demonstration shows the movement the user needs to focus on, such as wrist flexion or finger extension, thereby enhancing motor imagery through visual stimulation.

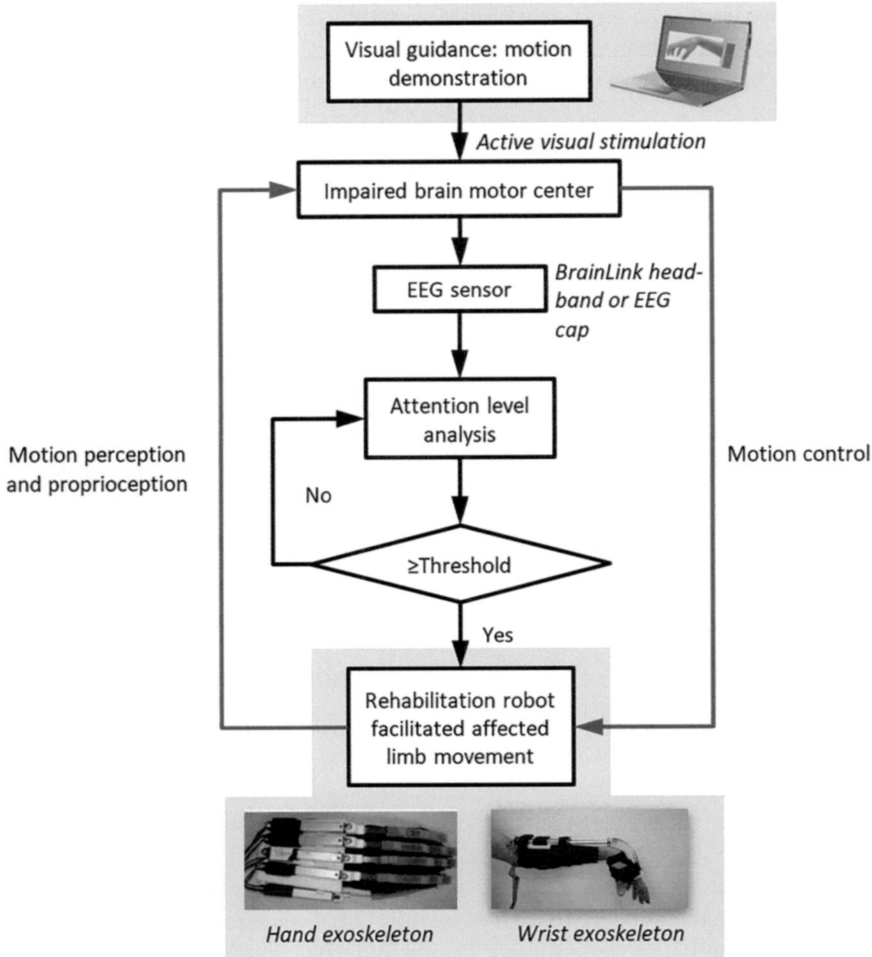

Fig. 5.1 Concept of brain-controlled hand and wrist rehabilitation based on attention level with visual guidance

The user interacts with the system by concentrating on the motion displayed on the screen and imagining performing the movement themselves. As the user's focus level rises, measured by the EEG sensor, it triggers the device once a predefined attention threshold is reached. This attention threshold functions as an activation switch for the exoskeleton, initiating the rehabilitation motion that matches the demonstrated movement. By enabling the user's focused mental engagement to activate the exoskeleton, the system not only supports active training but also helps patients regain control over specific wrist and hand movements by reinforcing neural pathways associated with those actions.

The dual stimulation provided by this design—visual guidance for mirror neuron activation and proprioceptive feedback from the exoskeleton—facilitates both active and passive forms of co-stimulation, which are essential for motor recovery. This coordinated approach is aimed at encouraging neuroplasticity through repetitive, attention-driven movements, which can help rebuild motor function in patients with impaired hand and wrist mobility. By simplifying the process with an attention-based threshold rather than complex motor imagery protocols, this design provides an accessible and effective rehabilitation solution for clinical and at-home use. The following sections provide an in-depth discussion of the hand and wrist exoskeleton design and the attention-based brain-controlled switching mechanism.

5.3 Hand and Wrist Exoskeletons

Hand Exoskeleton

In this study, the hand exoskeleton used the same structure that was mentioned in Chap. 4. A multi-segment hand exoskeleton was developed to support finger flexion and extension. Each finger is equipped with a dedicated actuator, allowing isolated movement control. This structure uses a flexible multi-segment mechanism attached to a steel strap and driven by a single linear motor per finger, achieving a highly adaptable fit that mitigates joint misalignment issues. Each actuator includes a spring layer that bends and moves in conjunction with the linear motor's motion, enabling the structure to mimic a circular sector as it follows the natural curvature of the fingers during movement.

The hand exoskeleton consists of five actuators—one per finger—secured to a fabric glove using Velcro straps, allowing easy replacement and custom fitting for various hand sizes. Each actuator's steel strap attaches to the motor via a compact 3D-printed connector, providing secure transmission of the linear motor's force to the fingers. The motors are mounted on a rigid part fixed to the forearm, ensuring stability and alignment across all actuators during use. To enhance comfort, the segments of the multi-segment mechanism were carefully designed, with segment thicknesses varying to match the finger joints' natural bending. Specifically, the segments positioned above the interphalangeal (IP) and metacarpophalangeal (MP) joints are thinner than those above the finger's proximal, distal, and middle phalanges, improving adaptability to finger motion. The segments for the thumb and other fingers vary in thickness to match each finger's unique range of motion, with segment dimensions optimized for smooth, controlled finger movement across the hand.

The hand exoskeleton's entire assembly, including the glove, actuators, and motors, weighs only 401 g, well below the target weight of 0.5 kg. The finger actuator segments were fabricated using VisiJet Crystal material for added flexibility and durability, while the motor attachment base was printed in PLA to provide a rigid foundation for the glove-mounted actuators.

Wrist Exoskeleton

As shown in Fig. 5.2a, the wrist exoskeleton is a modular design comprising five main components: two linear motors, a forearm support frame, connecting components, a hand support structure, and a pair of steel spring strips. These components are carefully aligned to control the wrist's extension, flexion, and ulnar/radial deviation through coordinated motor action. The forearm and hand are secured within the structure using adjustable support frames that keep the device stable during operation and minimize slippage.

Actuation is provided by two L12-100-100-6-I linear motors (Actuonix Motion Devices Inc., Canada), each capable of delivering a maximum force of 42 N and a stroke length of 100 mm. These motors engage the steel spring strips—each 120 mm in length, 8 mm in width, and 0.3 mm thick (65Mn steel)—to generate and transmit

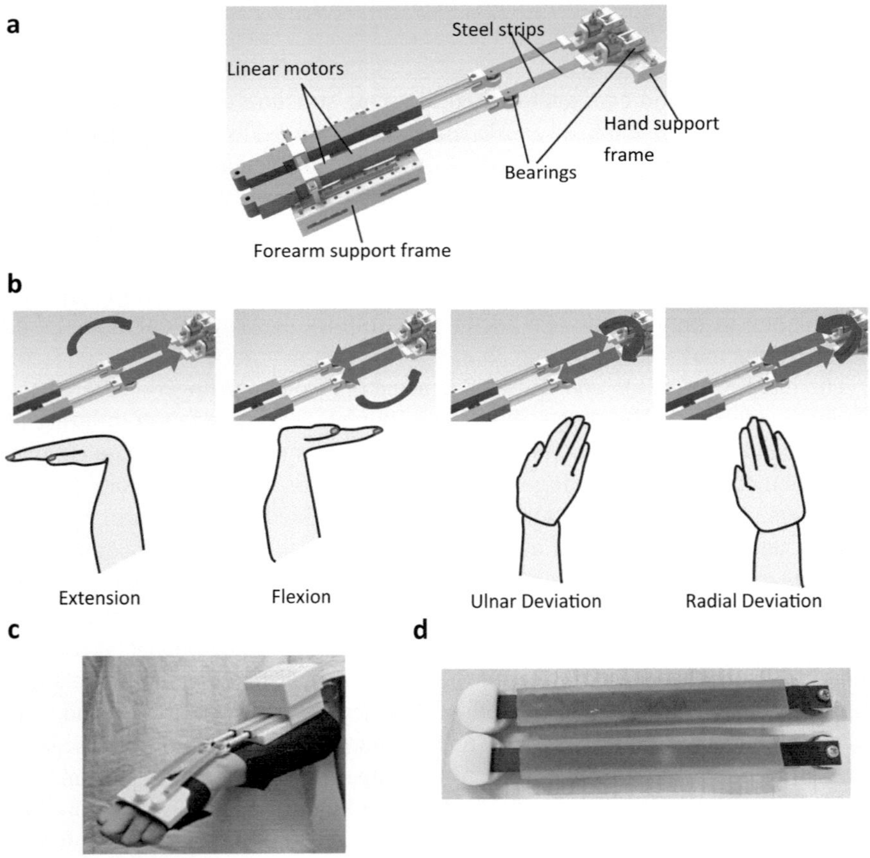

Fig. 5.2 Design of the wrist exoskeleton: **a** design, **b** movements, **c** the assembly, and **d** the silicone sheath enclosing the steel strip

force to the wrist. Different combinations of motor elongation produce targeted wrist motions; for example, varying the extension levels of the two strips allows precise control over ulnar and radial deviation, as illustrated in Fig. 5.2b. Bearings placed at connection points ensure smooth motion by allowing rotational flexibility where the spring strips connect to the motor and hand support frame. These connector bearings, designed for ease of attachment, prevent wear and improve the longevity and stability of the device. The forearm support frame has trapezoidal grooves that securely hold the motors in place while conforming to the natural contours of the arm, ensuring that the motors remain parallel for even actuation.

The wrist exoskeleton was constructed primarily from lightweight, 3D-printed polylactic acid (PLA), resulting in a device that weighs just 259 g (or 415 g including the controller), making it comfortable for extended wear. For user safety and comfort, the wrist exoskeleton's steel spring strips are encased in a silicone rubber jacket (1 mm thick) to prevent contact with the sharp steel edges. Additionally, the wearable structure was designed with fabric and Velcro adjustments to ensure a secure fit for a range of hand sizes. Velcro straps enable users to adjust the device across the forearm and thumb, accommodating both the conical shape of the arm and varying hand dimensions for a snug fit without pressure points.

In this study, this steel strip-driven wrist exoskeleton is used. It is worth mentioning that we introduced the multi-segment mechanism presented in Chap. 4 to the wrist exoskeleton in our previous study (Yang et al. 2021). With the multi-segment mechanism, the exoskeleton achieves the same functional range of motion (ROM) with less motor movement than the wrist exoskeleton shown in this chapter. Moreover, it can achieve three-DOF movements. The exoskeleton structure is illustrated in Fig. 5.3. One end of the multi-segment structure is connected to the linear motor's linkage via a bearing tray, while the other end is perpendicularly attached to the dorsal hand plate through a bearing block. The bearing block incorporates two vertically positioned bearings, forming a universal joint structure. The wrist exoskeleton achieves three-DOF movements through different stroke combinations of the actuators. When the multi-segment continuous structure is secured to the motor using Velcro, it bends and extends along with the motor's movement. Specifically, simultaneous forward or backward motion of both linear motors enables wrist flexion/extension. Conversely, when one motor moves forward while the other moves backward, the exoskeleton performs pronation/supination. When the multi-segment structure is detached, it moves forward and backward along with an elastic steel sheet, creating a parallelogram mechanism with the two parallel continuous structures. In this configuration, if one motor advances while the other remains stationary, the exoskeleton achieves radial/ulnar deviation.

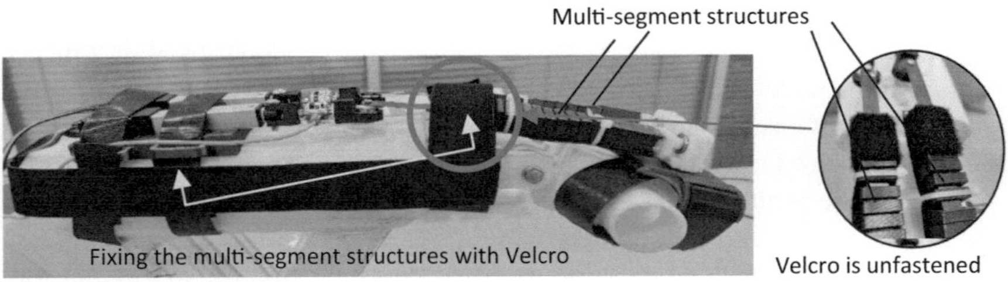

Fig. 5.3 A wrist exoskeleton with multi-segment structures

5.4 Attention-Controlled Switch for the Hand and Wrist Exoskeletons

The brain-actuated switch for the hand and wrist exoskeletons relies on real-time monitoring of the user's brain activity via EEG signals, captured using the the Brainlink Lite headset (Macrotellect Ltd., Shenzhen, China). This low-cost, lightweight device integrates three dry electrodes—a signal channel, a ground point (GND), and a reference point (REF)—into a convenient headband. The Brainlink Lite records EEG signals across several frequency bands, each corresponding to different status of consciousness:

- Delta (δ) (0.5–3.5 Hz): Associated with sleep.
- Theta (θ) (3.5–7.5 Hz): Linked to inefficiency and daydreaming.
- Alpha (α) (7.5–12 Hz): Reflects relaxation and inner peace.
- Beta (β) (12–30 Hz): Indicates heightened concentration and focus.
- Gamma (γ) (31 Hz and above): Represents attention and higher cognitive functions (Larsen and Wang 2011; Hammond 2007, 2011).

Using the attention level derived from these brain signals, the device determines whether the user is sufficiently focused to activate the exoskeleton. The exoskeleton operates in two states: *triggered* or *not triggered*. A threshold-based control principle governs this functionality:

$$f = \begin{cases} 1, AtL \geq AtL_{thr}(\text{exoskeleton triggered}) \\ 0, AtL < AtL_{thr}(\text{exoskeleton not triggered}) \end{cases} \tag{5.1}$$

where f is the control function, AtL represents the attention level, and AtL_{thr} represents the predefined threshold.

The Brainlink Lite is well-suited for rehabilitation due to its dry-electrode design, which eliminates the need for conductive gels. Its ThinkGear AM (TGAM) module quantifies the user's attention levels on a scale of 1 to 100 based on EEG data. When the attention level exceeds the threshold, the system activates the exoskeleton via the brain-controlled switch, encouraging active user participation in rehabilitation.

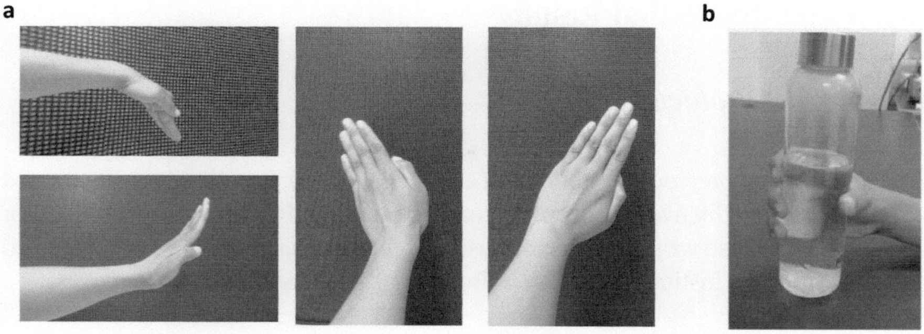

Fig. 5.4 Video demonstration of **a** four wrist movements and **b** hand grasping motion

The device also monitors the electrode–skin contact and provides warnings if EEG signals are poor, prompting adjustments to ensure reliable operation.

To enhance motor imagery, the system features a graphical user interface (GUI) built using MATLAB, which includes motion demonstrations. The GUI displays specific rehabilitation movements, such as wrist flexion or hand grasping, to guide the user in focusing and imagining the motion (see Fig. 5.4). This process leverages mirror neurons, which strengthen neural pathways by linking observed and imagined actions, thereby promoting motor recovery.

The GUI comprises three components: (a) a motion selection area for choosing the target movement; (b) a motion demonstration area displaying videos of the selected movement; (c) a real-time attention level bar showing the user's focus. When the attention level of the user surpasses the threshold, the exoskeleton is then activated by the brain-controlled switch, performing the selected motion and providing proprioceptive feedback. This feedback reinforces the connection between mental focus and physical movement, essential for effective rehabilitation.

The Brainlink Lite transmits data to MATLAB via Bluetooth, enabling real-time attention monitoring. An Arduino MEGA 2560 microcontroller interfaces with the exoskeleton's linear actuators, controlling their movements based on the user's focus. The Arduino's 0–5 V interface ensures consistent and reliable actuation, with predetermined movement amplitudes simplifying operation. This user-friendly system integrates cognitive and physical engagement, offering an accessible, cost-effective solution for both clinical and home-based rehabilitation.

The ThinkGear AM module integrated within the device samples EEG signals at a rate of 512 Hz (NeuroSky 2019). Then, attention values are calculated at a rate of 1 Hz based on the EEG band power values obtained from the Brainlink Lite software. Error checking was conducted for each data frame, with any frames containing errors being discarded. During experiments, occasional data loss was observed during transmission over the Bluetooth connection. On average, approximately 55 to 58 data points were successfully received in one minute. Since the threshold-based hand exoskeleton triggering does not require precise timing of attention data points, the data loss is not deemed significant for the exoskeleton control.

5.5 Experiments and Results

Experiment Protocols

As detailed in our previouse studies (Li et al. 2019a, 2019b), experiments were carried out to assess the effectiveness of the attention value-based switching mechanism for controlling hand and wrist exoskeletons using human participants. The study received approval from the Institutional Review Board of Xi'an Jiaotong University.

Attention Threshold Experiments

Determining an appropriate attention level threshold is critical for the proposed system. If the exoskeleton activates without sufficient user focus, active rehabilitation cannot be achieved. Conversely, overly high thresholds may reduce the user's motivation. Thus, experiments were designed to investigate suitable thresholds for the attention-based control system used in wrist and hand rehabilitation.

Hand experiments

As presented in our previouse study (Li et al. 2019b), the hand experiments involved 14 participants (10 males, 4 females, average age: 23.8, SD = 0.89), all with normal vision and neurological health. Conducted in a quiet room, participants wore the BrainLink device and sat in front of a laptop. The experiments measured attention levels under four conditions:

- **Concentration with Visual Guidance:** Participants watched a hand grasping video repeatedly for 50 s and focused on the motion.
- **Concentration without Visual Guidance:** Participants viewed a text prompt and imagined a grasping motion for 50 s without video aid.
- **Resting State:** Participants remained at rest, without engaging in any motor imagery, for 50 s.
- **Distraction:** Participants simultaneously watched three unrelated video clips, listened to noise (e.g., factory sounds), and answered random questions.

Each condition was repeated three times per participant, with attention levels recorded. Before testing, participants completed one trial to familiarize themselves with the process, and a two-minute break was provided between trials. Figure 5.5a illustrates the procedure.

Wrist experiments

As presented in our previouse study (Li et al. 2019a), twelve participants (7 males, 5 females, average age: 23.2, range: 22–25) participated in wrist experiments, conducted similarly to the hand experiments. Three experimental conditions were tested:

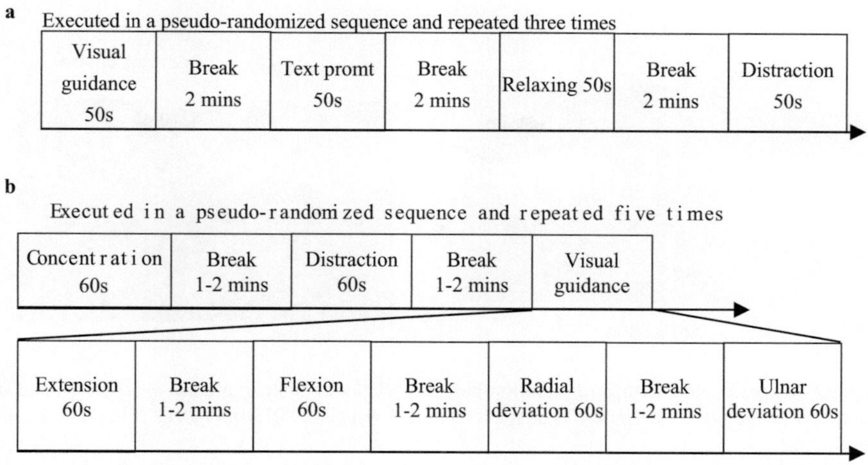

Fig. 5.5 Procedure of the attention threshold experiment: **a** comparison of relaxation, distraction, text prompt of imagining a grasping motion, and visual guidance of imagining a grasping motion, **b** comparison of distraction, focus on a static user interface with no motion displayed, and focus on video demonstrations of wrist movements (extension, flexion, radial deviation, and ulnar deviation). Combined and reformatted from our previous works (Li et al. 2019a, 2019b). (Li et al. 2019a) © 2019 IEEE. Used wit permission; (Li et al. 2019b) published under a Creative Commons CC-BY license

- **Distraction:** Participants experienced interruptions, such as movies, music, and random questions.
- **Concentration:** Participants concentrated on a static user interface with no motion displayed.
- **Concentration with Visual Guidance:** Participants focused on video demonstrations of wrist motions (extension, flexion, radial deviation, and ulnar deviation).

Each condition lasted one minute, with a 1–2 min break between trials. Trials were repeated five times in a pseudo-random order, and attention levels were recorded from 30-s stable periods. Figure 5.5b shows the procedure.

Attention-Based Control of the Exoskeletons

Hand experiments

As decribed in our previouse study (Li et al. 2019b), this experiment evaluated the success rate and reaction time of the attention-based hand exoskeleton control. Using thresholds determined in the attention threshold experiment, participants viewed a hand-grasping demonstration video and imagined performing the same motion (Fig. 5.6a).

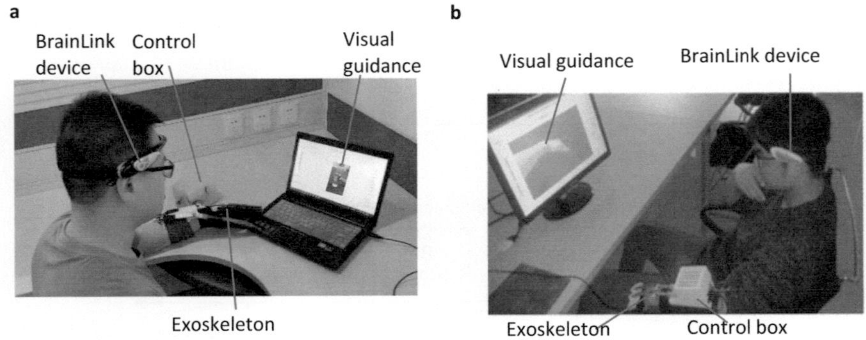

Fig. 5.6 Experimental set-ups of attention-based exoskeleton control: **a** hand exoskeleton and **b** wrist exoskeleton (the subfigure **b** is adapted from Ref. (Li et al. 2019a), © 2019 IEEE. Used with permission)

- **Customized Thresholds:** Set based on each participant's average attention level from the threshold experiment.
- **General Threshold:** Set as the average attention level across all participants.

The exoskeleton activated if the participant's attention exceeded the threshold. Participants repeated the process 20 times, with a 30-s time limit per trial. Trials exceeding the limit were marked as failures. Figure 5.7a outlines the procedure.

Wrist experiments

As demonstrated in our previouse work (Li et al. 2019a), wrist exoskeleton experiments followed similar protocols (Fig. 5.6b), focusing on one movement (extension)

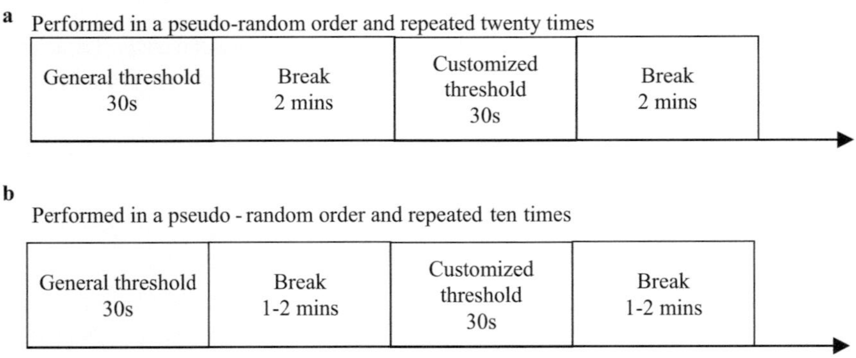

Fig. 5.7 The procedure of attention-based control of the exoskeletons experiment: **a** comparison between a fixed attention threshold and individually customized thresholds controlling the hand exoskeleton and **b** comparison between a fixed attention threshold and individually customized thresholds controlling the wrist exoskeleton. Combined and reformatted from our previous works (Li et al. 2019a, 2019b). Li et al. (2019a) © 2019 IEEE. Used with permission; (Li et al. 2019b) published under a Creative Commons CC-BY license

for simplicity. Participants viewed a wrist motion video and imagined performing the same motion. Customized and general thresholds were applied, as in the hand experiments. Attention levels were recorded, and the time to threshold and success rate were analyzed.

Each trial had a 30-s time limit, with 1–2 min breaks between trials. The process was repeated 10 times in a pseudo-random order. Figure 5.7b illustrates the procedure.

After the experiments, participants rated the system on a scale of 1–10 based on: (a) response speed: the time needed to react to changes in the attention level of the user; (b) accuracy: the system's ability to reflect attention levels correctly; (c) intuitiveness: the ease and convenience of the attention-based control. This feedback helped assess the usability and practicality of the proposed system.

Experiment Results

Attention Threshold Experiments

Hand Experiments

An average attention level was computed based on a 30-s data segment once the attention level had stabilized. The total sample size was 42, consisting of 14 subjects performing 3 repetitions each. As shown in Fig. 5.8, the mean attention values for the different experimental conditions were as follows: distraction (26.3 ± 10.7), relaxation (40.2 ± 10.7), concentration without visual guidance (76.4 ± 8.74), and concentration with visual guidance (81.1 ± 9.38). Normality testing was carried out using the Shapiro–Wilk method, with the results showing that the attention values for all experimental conditions followed a normal distribution: relaxation (W and p were 0.988 and 0.925, respectively), concentration without visual guidance (W and p were 0.981 and 0.7, respectively), distraction (W and p were 0.951 and 0.067, respectively), and concentration with visual guidance (W and p were 0.963 and 0.192, respectively). Then, a Levene's test for homogeneity of variances indicated no significant differences with $p = 0.734 > 0.05$, suggesting that the data variances were equal across groups.

Subsequently, a one-way ANOVA was conducted to test for significant differences among the experimental conditions. The results showed significant differences between groups ($p = 1.71 \times 10^{-67} < 0.05$). Post-hoc pairwise comparisons using a Student's t-test with Bonferroni correction were performed with R Project for Statistical Computing. The result showed that the distraction condition had significantly lower attention values than the other three conditions. The p values were 9.31×10^{-8} and $< 2.2 \times 10^{-16}$ when compared to relaxation and concentration with visual guidance, respectively. A significant difference was also found between the attention values in concentration conditions involving visual guidance and no visual guidance

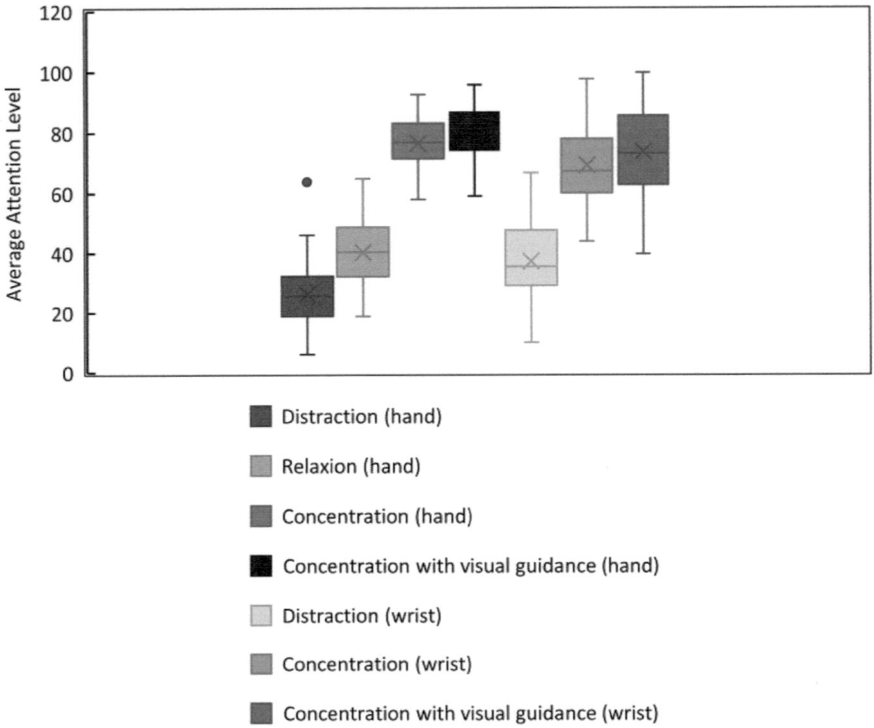

Fig. 5.8 Results of the attention threshold experiments for hand grasping and wrist movements. Data combined and reformatted from our previous works (Li et al. 2019a, 2019b). Li et al. (2019a) © 2019 IEEE. Used with permission; (Li et al. 2019b) published under a Creative Commons CC-BY license

($p = 4.96 \times 10^{-3}$). Lastly, the relaxation condition had significantly lower attention values than both the concentration conditions (involving visual guidance and no visual guidance) ($p < 2.2 \times 10^{-16}$).

Wrist experiments

For each trial, the mean attention level was computed from 30 s of data once the attention value reached a stable state. The attention values observed during motion demonstrations that utilized visual guidance are presented in Fig. 5.9. The average attention levels achieved with visual guidance during flexion, extension, ulnar deviation, and radial deviation were 77 ± 11.5, 74 ± 14.2, 79 ± 10.6, and 80 ± 10.3, respectively. A total of 60 observations were collected from 12 subjects, each contributing 5 repeated measurements. The Shapiro–Wilk test was conducted to assess normality of the data, using a significance threshold of 0.05. The results demonstrated that the attention levels associated with each movement conformed to a normal distribution. The W values for flexion, extension, ulnar deviation, and radial deviation were determined to be 0.977, 0.977, 0.970, and 0.961, respectively. Meanwhile, the corresponding p values were 0.315, 0.309, 0.151, and 0.051, respectively. A Levene's test revealed a violation of the assumption of homogeneity of variance ($p = 0.021$). Consequently, a Kruskal–Wallis test was performed to assess if there were any significant differences between the movements, which revealed no significant differences among these movements with $p = 0.079$.

Given the absence of significant differences in attention levels between flexion, extension, ulnar deviation, and radial deviation under visual guidance, extension was selected as the representative motion for comparison against the "concentration without visual guidance" and "distraction" conditions. As shown in Fig. 5.8, the mean attention levels for the focusing, distraction, and focusing with visual guidance conditions were 69 ± 13.1, 37 ± 11.8, and 74 ± 14.2, respectively. A Shapiro–Wilk test was conducted to ascertain the normality of distribution for attention levels across each condition. The results were as follows: for the concentration condition, $W = 0.967$ with a p-value of 0.108; in the distraction condition, $W = 0.984$ and $p = 0.604$; and for the concentration with visual guidance condition, $W = 0.976$ and $p = 0.283$. Then a Levene's test confirmed equal variances with $p = 0.232$. Accordingly, a one-way ANOVA was conducted to assess whether there were statistically significant differences among the three conditions, and the results showed significant differences ($p = 7.79 \times 10^{-37} < 0.05$). Pairwise comparisons were conducted using a Student's t-test with Bonferroni correction. The distraction condition showed significantly lower attention levels than the concentration and concentration with visual guidance conditions ($p = 7.83 \times 10^{-23} < 0.05/3$, $p = 2.12 \times 10^{-26} < 0.05/3$). Additionally, a significant difference was observed between the focusing with visual guidance and concentration without visual guidance conditions ($p = 5.84 \times 10^{-3} < 0.05/3$). These results indicate that participants exhibited higher attention levels when concentration with visual guidance compared to concentration without visual guidance.

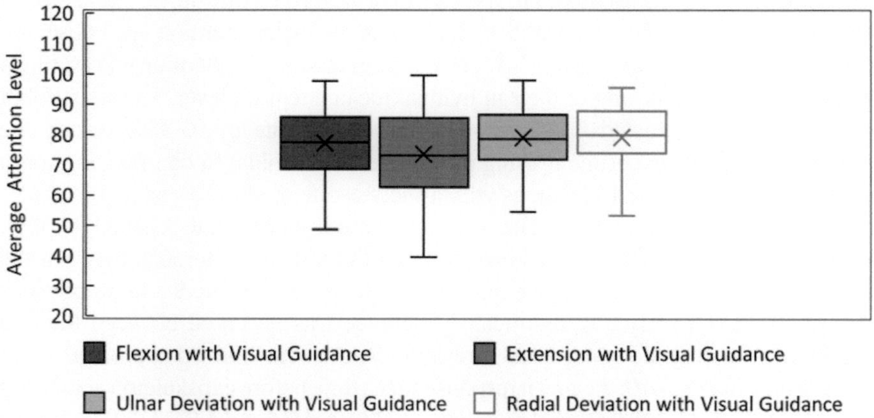

Fig. 5.9 Comparison of four wrist movements in the attention threshold experiment for wrist movements. Adapted from Li et al. (2019a) © 2019 IEEE. Used with permission

Attention-Based Control of the Exoskeletons

Hand experiments

A total of 14 subjects participated in the experiment, with each subject performing 20 trials. An attention level threshold of 81 was set based on the mean attention level obtained in the experiment. Additionally, a personalized attention threshold was established for each participant based on their individual average attention level. The hand exoskeleton attained a total success rate of 94.64% when using customized thresholds, while using the generalized threshold, the success rate increased to 96.43%. Overall, the system achieved an actuation success rate of 95.54%. The results of the ANOVA indicated no significant differences in actuation performance between the generalized and customized thresholds with $p = 0.48 > 0.05$. It should be noted that the actuation success rates—whether based on customized or general thresholds—were found to be non-normally distributed according to the Shapiro–Wilk test. The test yielded $p < 0.001$ for the general threshold and $p = 0.002$ for the customized threshold, respectively. Additionally, Levene's test indicated heterogeneous variances ($p = 0.045 < 0.05$), suggesting a violation of the assumption of homogeneity of variance.

As shown in Fig. 5.10, the average delay before activation was 8.06 ± 6.15 s for the general threshold and 8.08 ± 6.21s for the customized threshold. The Shapiro–Wilk test revealed non-normal distribution of activation times for both the general and customized thresholds (general: $W = 0.798$, $p < 2.2 \times 10^{-16}$; customized: $W = 0.838$, $p = 5.639 \times 10^{-16}$). Consequently, a Mann–Whitney U test was employed to assess differences in activation times between the two conditions. The difference in activation time was not significant ($U = 34{,}734$, $p = 0.561$).

Wrist experiments

The sample size consisted of 120 trials (12 subjects × 10 repetitions). A generalized attention level threshold was established based on the mean attention level observed in the experiment (attention level: 74). The participant-specific attention level settings were determined according to their individual mean attention level. The wrist robot was successfully actuated 112 times with a success rate of 93.33% during the exoskeleton control experiment using customized thresholds. In contrast, the robot was successfully actuated 116 times with a success rate of 96.67%) using the generalized attention level threshold. The overall actuation success rate reached 95.00%. Afterwards, Wilson score intervals were applied to test the difference between the two proportions, with a confidence interval of 0.029 and a difference in proportions (Δp) of 0.033 ($CI < \Delta p$). A significant difference was observed between the two conditions, favoring the generalized threshold over the customized approach.

As shown in Fig. 5.10, the mean response time (time before exoskeleton actuation) was 4.62 ± 4.98 s for the general attention level threshold and 4.04 ± 4.08 s for the customized attention level threshold. To assess the normality of the acquired data, a Shapiro–Wilk test was conducted. The results revealed that the response times under both experimental conditions did not adhere to a normal distribution. In the

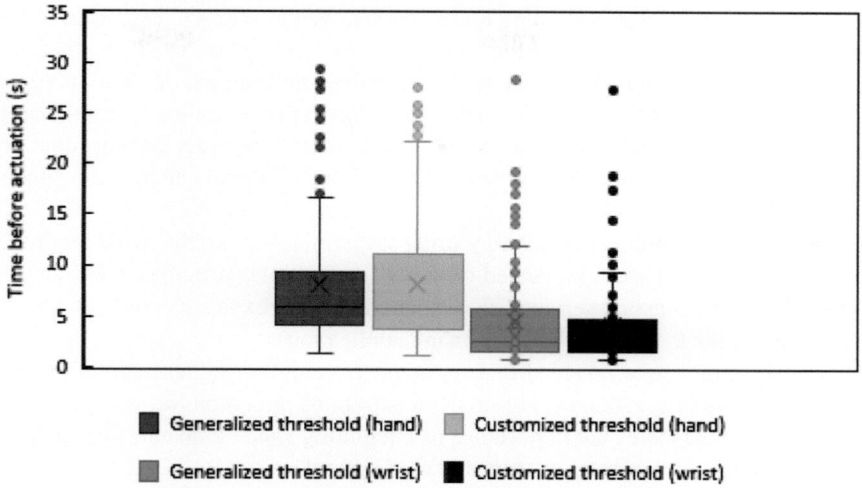

Fig. 5.10 Response time of the attention-based hand and wrist exoskeleton control. Data combined and reformatted from our previous works (Li et al. 2019a, 2019b). Li et al. (2019a) © 2019 IEEE. Used with permission; (Li et al. 2019b) published under a Creative Commons CC-BY license

focusing condition, the Shapiro–Wilk test yielded $W = 0.703$ ($p = 2.897 \times 10^{-13}$); in the distraction condition, $W = 0.984$ ($p = 0.604$); and in the focusing with visual guidance condition, $W = 0.725$ ($p = 8.677 \times 10^{-13}$). Consequently, a Mann–Whitney U test was conducted to compare the differences in response times between the two conditions. The results showed no significant difference in response time between the two experimental conditions ($W = 5431.5$, $p = 0.764$).

5.6 Discussion and Conclusion

Discussion

The proposed robotic mechanism for the wrist exoskeleton successfully combines rigidity and flexibility, achieving effective rehabilitation while maintaining a cost-effective design. Unlike traditional EEG-based wrist exoskeletons (Coffey et al. 2014), our system employs low-cost devices to facilitate four distinct wrist motions. This accessibility enhances its suitability for both rehabilitation centers and home-based use. Additionally, compared to a prior wrist exoskeleton with similar mechanical structures (Higuma et al. 2018), our system incorporates BCI control in a closed-loop configuration, which improves patient engagement and rehabilitation outcomes.

The wrist exoskeleton, including the controller, weighs 415 g (259 g without the controller). During experiments, the controller was mounted on participants' forearms. However, for clinical applications, placing the controller on a surface such as a table is recommended to reduce the arm's load, especially for patients experiencing muscle weakness. Future iterations of the design should consider adding force or/and posture sensors to improve human–robot collaboration and enhance movement assistance.

One notable limitation observed during experiments was the wear on EEG sensor electrodes caused by repeated cleaning for multiple participants. While this issue reduces the sensor's service life compared to more expensive alternatives, its affordability offsets this drawback for many applications.

Experimental results revealed that participants achieved higher attention levels when visual guidance, such as motion demonstrations on a monitor, was provided. This finding underscores the importance of integrating visual guidance into rehabilitation training to enhance user focus and engagement.

Regarding system evaluation, no significant differences in activation time were observed between using general and customized attention thresholds. However, the general threshold yielded slightly better success rates, likely due to some customized thresholds being set too high and becoming unattainable. These results suggest that a general attention threshold offers a practical and efficient solution for exoskeleton control, simplifying the process without compromising performance.

Future research should explore demographic factors, such as age and gender, that may influence attention levels. Tailoring attention thresholds based on these factors could enable more personalized rehabilitation experiences, addressing the specific needs and impairments of individual patients.

While the proposed attention-based control solution actively engages users in their rehabilitation process, further studies are needed to investigate the synchronization of active movement intentions, derived from EEG signals, with passive rehabilitation provided by the exoskeleton. Combining sEMG and EEG signals has the potential to decode hand motion more effectively and extend the scope of active rehabilitation training sessions (Yang et al. 2021, 2022).

It is worth noting that this study primarily involved young, healthy participants, which limits the generalizability of the findings. Future experiments should include participants with stroke-related impairments to validate the system's clinical applicability.

Linking movement intentions with sensorimotor feedback shows significant promise for stroke rehabilitation. By using attention values as input commands for the hand exoskeleton, this approach simplifies the control process, making it more practical and affordable compared to other costly and complex BCI methods.

Conclusion

In this chapter, we introduce attention-controlled hand and wrist rehabilitation systems using an affordable EEG sensor. The proposed solution is user-friendly and cost-effective, making it suitable for both clinical and home-based rehabilitation. Two key innovations of this study include using attention-based control to enhance patient engagement in robotic-based rehabilitation and augment attention levels with visual guidance.

The experimental results demonstrated that participants achieved higher attention values when visual guidance was provided during motion demonstrations. The average activation success rate of the attention-based switch exceeded 95%, confirming the system's reliability. Furthermore, the system evaluation revealed no significant difference in activation time between general and customized attention thresholds. These findings indicate that a general attention threshold is a practical and effective choice for hand exoskeleton activation, simplifying the setup process without reducing performance.

Future research should focus on conducting clinical trials with stroke patients to validate the system's therapeutic efficacy and feasibility in real-world scenarios. Additionally, further refinement of the design and integration of advanced control algorithms could enhance the system's usability and expand its applications in stroke rehabilitation.

References

Carmeli E, Peleg S, Bartur G et al (2011) HandTutor enhanced hand rehabilitation after stroke—a pilot study. Physiother Res Int 16:191–200. https://doi.org/10.1002/pri.485

Coffey AL, Leamy DJ, Ward TE (2014) A novel BCI-controlled pneumatic glove system for home-based neurorehabilitation. In: 2014 36th annual international conference of the IEEE engineering in medicine and biology society. EMBC, pp 3622–3625

Hammond DC (2007) What is neurofeedback? J Neurother. https://doi.org/10.1300/J184v10n04_04

Hammond DC (2011) What is neurofeedback: an update. J Neurother. https://doi.org/10.1080/10874208.2011.623090

Heo P, Gu GM, Lee S Jin et al (2012) Current hand exoskeleton technologies for rehabilitation and assistive engineering. Int J Precis Eng Manufact 13:807–824. https://doi.org/10.1007/s12541-012-0107-2

Higuma T, Kiguchi K, Arata J (2018) Low-profile two-degree-of-freedom wrist exoskeleton device using multiple spring blades. IEEE Robot Autom Lett 3:305–311

Jiang N, Dremstrup K, Farina D (2014) A novel brain-computer interface for chronic stroke. In: Brain-computer interface research, pp 51–61

Jiang N, Mrachacz-kersting N, Xu R et al (2014) An accurate , versatile , and robust brain switch for neurorehabilitation. In: Brain-computer interface research, pp 47–61

Johansson BB (2011) Current trends in stroke rehabilitation: a review with focus on brain plasticity. Acta Neurol Scand 123:147–159. https://doi.org/10.1111/j.1600-0404.2010.01417.x

Krebs HI, Volpe BT, Williams D et al (2007) Robot-aided neurorehabilitation: a robot for wrist rehabilitation. IEEE Trans Neural Syst Rehabil Eng 15:327–335. https://doi.org/10.1109/TNSRE.2007.903899

Kutner NG, Zhang R, Butler AJ et al (2010) Quality-of-life change associated with robotic-assisted therapy to improve hand motor function in patients with subacute stroke: a randomized clinical trial. Phys Ther 90:493–504. https://doi.org/10.2522/ptj.20090160

Larsen EA, Wang AI (2011) Classification of EEG signals in a brain-computer interface system. Norwegian University of Science and Technology. https://doi.org/10.1037/0022-3514.72.3.515

Li M, Xu G, Xie J, Chen C (2018) A review: motor rehabilitation after stroke with control based on human intent. Proc Inst Mech Eng H 232:344–360. https://doi.org/10.1177/0954411918755828

Li M, Liang Z, He B et al (2019a) Attention-controlled assistive wrist rehabilitation using a low-cost EEG sensor. IEEE Sens J 19:6497–6507. https://doi.org/10.1109/JSEN.2019.2910318

Li M, He B, Liang Z et al (2019b) An attention-controlled hand exoskeleton for the rehabilitation of finger extension and flexion using a rigid-soft combined mechanism. Front Neurorobot 13:1–13. https://doi.org/10.3389/fnbot.2019.00034

Maciejasz P, Eschweiler J, Gerlach-Hahn K et al (2014) A survey on robotic devices for upper limb rehabilitation. J Neuroeng Rehabil 11:3. https://doi.org/10.1186/1743-0003-11-3

NeuroSky (2019) TGAM1 characteristics. http://neurosky.com/biosensors/eeg-sensor/?tdsourcetag=s_pctim_aiomsg. Accessed 7 May 2019

Oztop E, Kawato M, Arbib MA (2013) Mirror neurons: functions, mechanisms and models. Neurosci Lett 540:43–55. https://doi.org/10.1016/j.neulet.2012.10.005

Squeri V, Masia L, Giannoni P et al (2013) Wrist rehabilitation in chronic stroke patients by means of adaptive, progressive robot aided therapy. In: IEEE Transactions on neural systems and rehabilitation engineering early ace, pp 312–325. https://doi.org/10.1109/TNSRE.2013.2250521

Takahashi CD, Der-Yeghiaian L, Le V et al (2008) Robot-based hand motor therapy after stroke. Brain 131:425–437. https://doi.org/10.1093/brain/awm311

Teo WP, Chew E (2014) Is motor-imagery brain-computer interface feasible in stroke rehabilitation? PM and R 6:723–728. https://doi.org/10.1016/j.pmrj.2014.01.006

Ueki S, Nishimoto Y, Abe M et al (2008) Development of virtual reality exercise of hand motion assist robot for rehabilitation therapy by patient self-motion control. In: 2008 30th annual international conference of the IEEE engineering in medicine and biology society. IEEE, pp 4282–4285

van Dokkum LEH, Ward T, Laffont I (2015) Brain computer interfaces for neurorehabilitation-its current status as a rehabilitation strategy post-stroke. Ann Phys Rehabil Med 58:3–8. https://doi.org/10.1016/j.rehab.2014.09.016

Wolf SL, Winstein CJ, Miller JP, Morris D (2015) Effect of constraint-induced movement therapy on upper extremity function 3 to 9 months after stroke. JAMA 296:2095–2104. https://doi.org/10.1001/jama.296.17.2095

Yang S, Li M, Wang J (2022) Fusing sEMG and EEG to increase the robustness of hand motion recognition using functional connectivity and GCN. IEEE Sens J 22:24309–24319. https://doi.org/10.1109/JSEN.2022.3221417

Yang S, Li M, Wang J et al (2021) A novel wrist rehabilitation exoskeleton using 3D-printed multi-segment mechanism. In: Proceedings of the annual international conference of the IEEE engineering in medicine and biology society, EMBS

Chapter 6
Leveraging Fingertip Cutaneous Haptic Stimulation to Enhance Attention in Exoskeleton-Based Hand Rehabilitation

Active participation during rehabilitation process leads to improved therapeutic results. This chapter describes the development of an exoskeleton-assisted hand therapy platform that integrates fingertip cutaneous haptic stimulation, the first attempt to combine these methods for enhancing training engagement. Using soft material 3D printing techniques, we developed low-cost, rapid-prototyped, and uniform-performance soft pneumatic actuators designed to deliver fingertip haptic sensations. The cutaneous stimulation delivered to the fingertip is synchronized with the movement generated by the hand exoskeleton. The force applied during the virtual grasp of a drinking glass was estimated using data from natural hand movements. System characterization experiments compared exoskeleton-supported hand motions under conditions with and without cutaneous stimulation at the fingertips in able-bodied participants. Participants' attention levels were assessed through EEG signals captured by the BrainLink headset. Results show that each haptic actuator is notably light, weighing approximately 6.8 g ($\pm$0.23 g) with stable performance and minimal hysteresis. The user study demonstrated significantly increased attention levels with added haptic stimulation, particularly when the grasping weight was heavier (300 g vs. 150 g). We conclude that fingertip haptic stimulation enhances user attention during exoskeleton-assisted hand exercises, potentially improving rehabilitation engagement.

6.1 Introduction

Hand rehabilitation typically involves continuous passive motion (CPM) exercises, where repetitive tasks like grasping improve hand strength, range of motion (ROM), and accuracy, often assisted by therapists or robotic devices (Ueki et al. 2012). Active involvement in rehabilitation training leads to better outcomes (Teo and Chew 2014; Ang and Guan 2013; Sagen et al. 2024). However, CPM exercises are passive,

M. Li and B. He, *Intention-Controlled Hand Rehabilitation for Stroke Survivors*,
https://doi.org/10.1007/978-981-95-4196-6_6

making it challenging for patients to stay engaged. Multi-modal sensory feedback can enrich rehabilitation experiences, enhancing motor learning, restoring the sensorimotor loop, and promoting functional recovery (Sigrist et al. 2013; Sharififar et al. 2018; Takeuchi and Izumi 2013). Previous studies have combined visual and auditory cues with rehabilitation training to increase engagement and motivation (Li et al. 2018; Cameirão et al. 2012; Yue et al. 2017; Secoli et al. 2011). Visual feedback helps track hand movements and improve task performance, while auditory cues support rhythmic movements and exercise duration (Song and Ryu 2016; Lee et al. 2018).

Stroke survivors often experience diminished haptic sensation in their hands (Heo et al. 2012), and haptic feedback during virtual reality-based rehabilitation has been shown to improve motor relearning (Piggott et al. 2016a). Hand exoskeletons can assist movement during CPM training and provide sensorimotor feedback. Cutaneous (or tactile) feedback, elicited through activation of cutaneous mechanoreceptors, helps sense when contact occurs and identify what the surface feels like (Lim et al. 2014). Pairing skin-level touch feedback with exoskeleton-supported rehabilitation training could simultaneously provide sensorimotor and tactile feedback, enhancing training involvement and promoting motor function restoration. This work marks the initial effort to merge cutaneous haptic stimulation with robotic exoskeleton support for hand therapy.

For effective integration, the haptic devices need to be lightweight, small, inexpensive, and comfortable. Fingertips are highly sensitive and frequently engage in contact interactions, making it more effective to deliver tactile feedback specifically to the fingertips rather than the entire hand. This targeted approach also helps minimize the dimensions and mass of the haptic device. Recent advancements in fingertip-mounted haptic feedback systems have focused on minimizing size and complexity (Pacchierotti et al. 2017; Schorr and Okamura 2017; Minamizawa et al. 2010; Zhai et al. 2021). Soft robotics offers a promising approach to delivering haptic feedback via wearable, soft devices. Previously, we developed a set of pneumatic actuators to enable simultaneous palpation across multiple fingers (Li et al. 2014a, 2014b), but traditional fabrication methods like casting and molding were costly and difficult to replicate consistently (Gul et al. 2018). With recent advances in 3D printing, we can now produce soft pneumatic actuators more affordably and efficiently (Gul et al. 2018; Yap et al. 2016; Ang and Yeow 2017).

This chapter draws upon our previous studies, where we introduced a hybrid rigid-soft mechanism designed for hand exoskeleton systems (Chap. 4). We now present fingertip-based cutaneous haptic feedback system integrated into an exoskeleton-supported hand rehabilitation platform. By integrating sensorimotor feedback from the exoskeleton with cutaneous haptic feedback, the rehabilitation process becomes more engaging, increasing patient focus during hand movement exercises. This study was first published in our previous article (Li et al. 2021), and in this chapter, we reorganize the methods and results for further clarity.

The layout of this chapter is structured in the following manner: Sect. 6.2 introduces the concept of integrating wearable exoskeleton technology with fingertip-based cutaneous haptics. Section 6.3 delves into the design and functionality of the fingertip cutaneous haptic stimulation system. Section 6.4 focuses on system integration and control mechanisms. Section 6.5 details the experimental protocol, followed by Sect. 6.6, which presents the experimental results. Finally, Sect. 6.7 discusses the findings and their implications.

6.2 Concept of Integration of Hand Exoskeleton and Fingertip Cutaneous Haptic Stimulation

Figure 6.1a presents the concept of our integrated system combining a hand exoskeleton with fingertip cutaneous haptic stimulation. In the conventional system, the hand exoskeleton assists the patient's fingers with passive flexion and extension movements during CPM therapy. These passive and repetitive exercises enhance hand function—such as ROM and grip strength—through the provision of sensorimotor feedback. However, due to the passive nature of the training, patients often struggle to stay focused and engaged.

To address this, we propose adding fingertip haptic feedback to enhance patient involvement. The hand exoskeleton, powered by linear motors, assists with finger flexion and extension, generating sensorimotor feedback. Meanwhile, fingertip-mounted haptic actuators provide additional tactile stimulation by creating contact forces, enhancing somatosensory feedback. By integrating haptic cues with robotic exoskeleton assistance, the system seeks to (a) enhance motor learning, (b) reestablish the sensory-motor integration pathway, and (c) facilitate the restoration of hand motor abilities, ultimately increasing patient engagement throughout the rehabilitation process.

6.3 Cutaneous Haptic Stimulation at the Fingertip

Researchers have developed actuators with air chambers and inflatable surfaces to produce tactile pressure at the fingertip through interaction with the actuator to deliver cutaneous haptic sensations (Lim et al. 2014; Li et al. 2014a, 2014b; Sarkar et al. 2020). These actuators were conventionally manufactured through casting and molding processes with materials like silicone rubber and PDMS (Lim et al. 2014; Li et al. 2014a, 2014b; Sarkar et al. 2020). These methods, however, involve high production costs and require significant time investment due to the need for new molds with each prototype iteration. The quality of prototypes can be difficult to control. To overcome these challenges, we adopted soft material 3D printing techniques, enabling faster, more cost-effective prototyping of flexible pneumatic devices that provide tactile feedback at the fingertips.

As shown in Fig. 6.1b, the developed actuator incorporates an air cavity, bounded by a top layer with a thickness of 0.45 mm, a 2.5 mm-thick oval sidewall and bottom

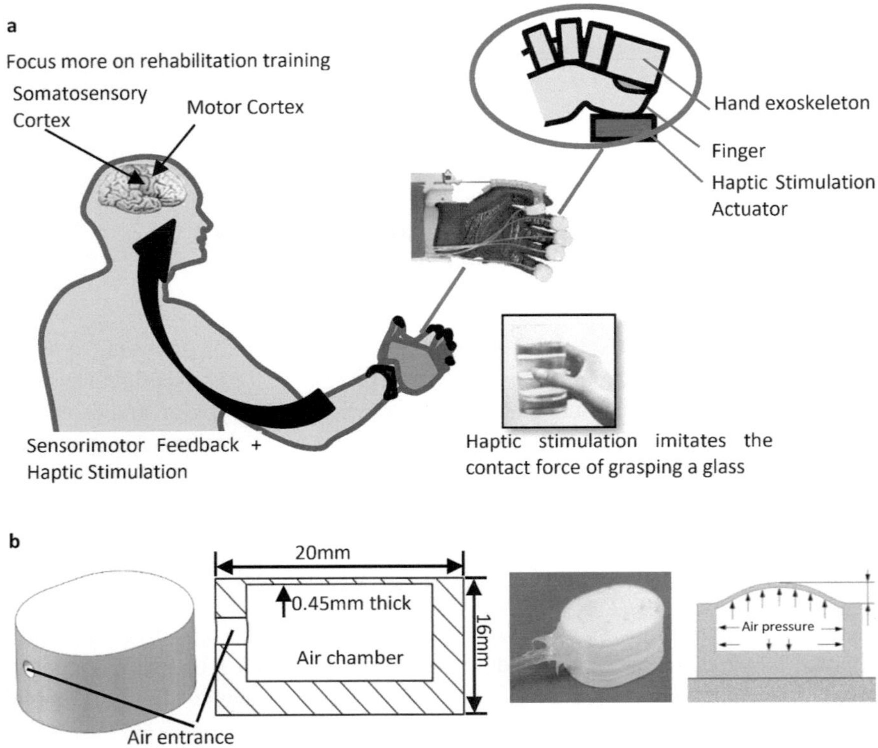

Fig. 6.1 Diagrams showcasing **a** our robotic hand rehabilitation solution that merges an exoskeleton with tactile stimulation at the fingertips and **b** the designed pneumatic actuator for haptic feedback. Reformatted from our previous works (Li et al. 2021), published under a Creative Commons CC-BY license

layer. This fingertip actuator was fabricated via 3D printing utilizing Ninjaflex, a flexible thermoplastic elastomer (NinjaTek 2019), on a Lulzbot TAZ 6 printer operating at a layer resolution of 0.15 mm. The chamber structures were printed without the need for support material; however, minor sagging was observed in the initial layers, although it had no discernible impact on the actuator's functionality. An air tubing (2 mm diameter) is attached to the actuator through clear silicone rubber adhesive (RTV 108) (Momentive 2020). Upon inflation of the chamber with air, the working surface expands, thereby enhancing the contact force at the fingertip interface, whereas minimal deformation occurs in the base and side structures The relationship between input pressure and contact force was calibrated through experiments outlined in Sects. 6.5.2 and 6.6.2. A 3D-printed fixture and Velcro served to secure the haptic actuator to the user's fingertip.

The hand exoskeleton directs the user's fingers through the grasping motion. As the exoskeleton performs bending and straightening motions, the fingertip haptic feedback intensity is modified to replicate the pressure felt when interacting with a virtual item, such as a glass container. Based on the exoskeleton's mechanical configuration, there is a linear correlation between the motor's displacement and the finger bending angle (Li et al. 2019). The displacement of the motor is measured using a stroke feedback signal obtained from a JY-DAM10AIAO analog I/O module (Beijing Elit Gathering Electron, China), which serves as the basis for calculating the corresponding finger joint angles.

When the finger approaches the simulated drinking glass, the haptic feedback actuator initiates operation. A glass-grasping model, derived from the experimental results presented in Sects. 6.5.1 and 6.6.1, is used to determine the target contact force for each fingertip. The required pressure for each actuator is then calculated from the desired contact force with the experimentally validated mapping from input pressure to resulting contact force, formulated in Eq. 6.1 (Sect. 6.6.2). An ITV0010 pressure regulator (SMC, Japan) receives the output signal (analog) for precise pressure adjustment, and an air pump from U-STAR (model U-STAR601, China) provides the needed air pressure.

6.4 System Consolidation and Control

Figure 6.2 illustrates the system consolidation and control for the hand rehabilitation system, which merges robotic exoskeleton support for hand motion with skin-based haptic stimulation. An Arduino Mega 2560 microcontroller is used to execute the predefined motor stroke sequence. Once a triggering command is sent from the host computer, the Arduino Mega 2560 sends commands to the linear motors of the hand exoskeleton. Then, the linear position feedback from the motor is directed to a JY-DAM10AIAO analog I/O module for signal acquisition and processing. Depending on the chosen mode and motor stroke feedback, the desired haptic force is computed and sent back to the same analog I/O module, which then adjusts the pneumatic pressure in cutaneous stimulation actuators at the fingertip through the pressure adjustment modules (SMC ITV0010). As previously outlined, compressed air is delivered using an air pump (U-STAR601). The system continuously monitors feedback signals from the pressure adjustment modules via the JY-DAM10AIAO module to ensure reliable operation.

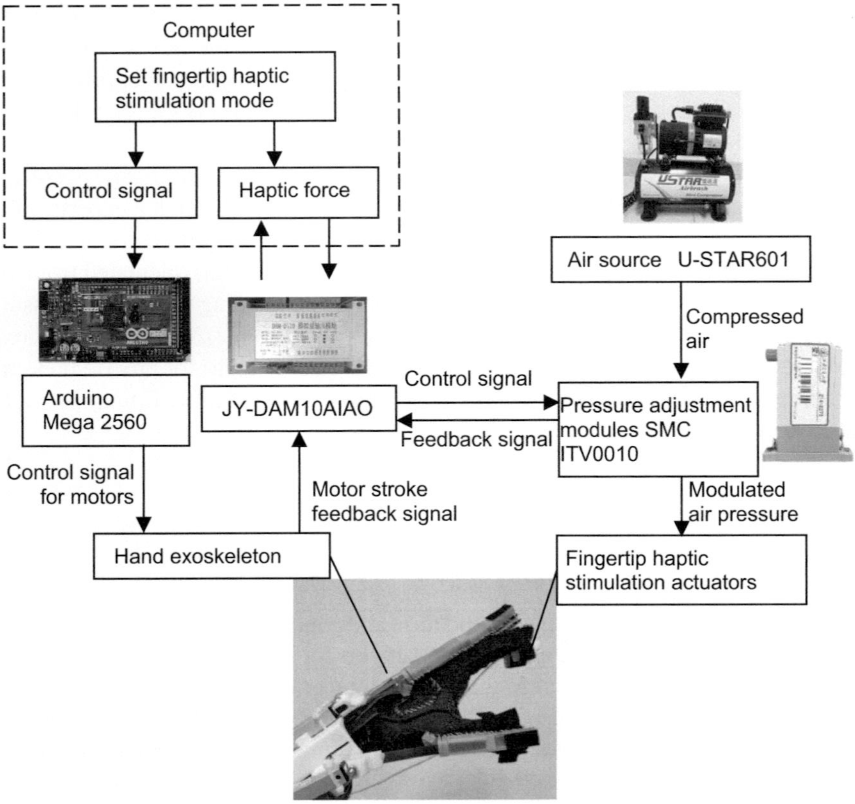

Fig. 6.2 Integration and control architecture of the hand rehabilitation system incorporating both a hand exoskeleton and fingertip haptic feedback mechanisms. Reformatted from our previous works (Li et al. 2021), published under a Creative Commons CC-BY 4.0 license

6.5 Experimental Setups and Protocols

Investigation of Fingertip Contact Force Changes During Glass Grasping

The variation in fingertip contact forces throughout the glass-grasping process was investigated through a controlled experiment. The resulting data were used to create a computational framework representing the interaction forces during glass grasping, intended for cutaneous haptic rendering based on the observed contact force patterns.

The experimental group consisted of ten individuals (seven men and three women, average age: 27), all of whom were right-handed. A 3D-printed replica of a glass (dimensions: 70 mm diameter × 120 mm height, weight: 150 g), equipped with embedded force sensors, was utilized as shown in Fig. 6.3. The object was made from

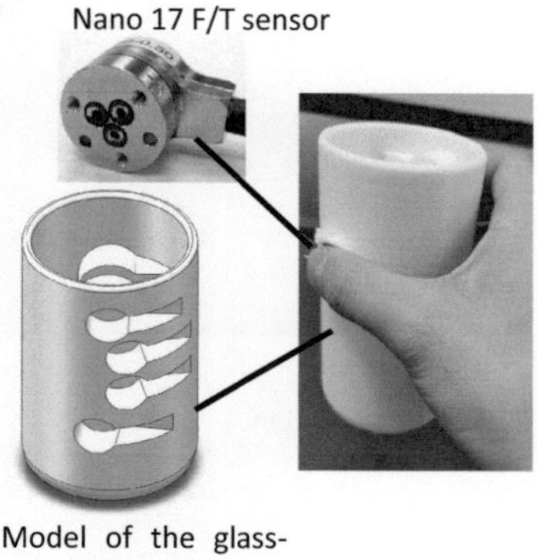

Fig. 6.3 Schematic and photograph of a sensor-integrated, 3D-printed glass-shaped object used in the experimental investigation of fingertip contact force evolution during grasping. Reformatted from our previous works (Li et al. 2021), published under a Creative Commons CC-BY 4.0 license

PLA material and featured five grooves to accommodate SI-12-0.12 force sensors (ATI Nano 17, USA), each assigned to a finger. The experimental setup included four different object masses (ranging from 150 to 300 g with an interval of 50 g), achieved by varying the amount of water inside the glass-shaped object. Participants were required to perform five trials per weight while maintaining a uniform grasping posture. Conducted under the ethical guidelines with the approval of the Institutional Review Board at Xi'an Jiaotong University, this study required all participants to provide written consent before participating.

Validation of System Performance and Assessment of Haptic Stimulation's Impact on User Attention

Technical Evaluation of the Haptic Actuation Mechanism and Stimulation Protocol

The mass of the haptic actuators for the five fingers was quantified using a high-precision electronic balance (measurement range: 0–100 g, resolution: 0.01 g). Additionally, the deformation behavior of the actuators was evaluated under different inflation pressure levels (0–100 kPa, with 0.5 kPa intervals). As shown in Fig. 6.4a, the HG-C1100 model from Panasonic, a precision laser displacement sensor manufactured in Japan was used to measure actuator deformation with an accuracy of 79 μm and a measurement range of ± 35 mm. The pressure was controlled via the same analog I/O module mentioned before (JY-DAM10AIAO), which sent signals to the pressure adjustment module (SMC ITV0010). The inflation and deflation of the actuators were repeated five times for each test cycle, lasting 100 s. Contact forces were calibrated during inflation and deflation between 0 and 100 kPa.

For force measurement, the SI-12-0.12 variant of the ATI Nano 17 sensor was affixed to a custom-designed contact block produced using Ninjaflex-based additive

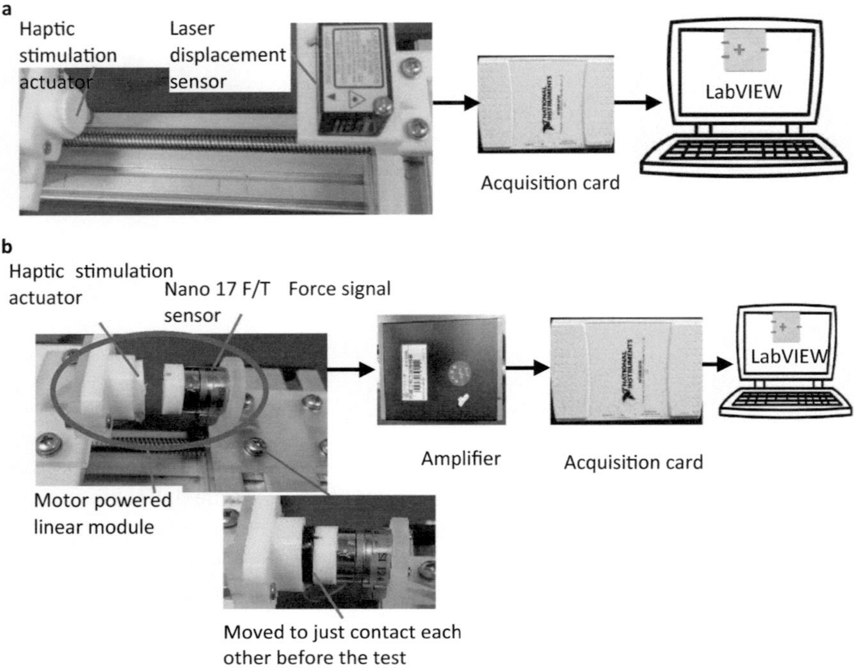

Fig. 6.4 Experimental setup illustrating **a** the deflection behavior and **b** the contact force generated by the actuator, haptic stimulation response. Reformatted from our previous works (Li et al. 2021), published under a Creative Commons CC-BY 4.0 license

Fig. 6.5 Configuration of the experimental system used to evaluate haptic stimulation response. Reformatted from our previous works (Li et al. 2021), published under a Creative Commons CC-BY license

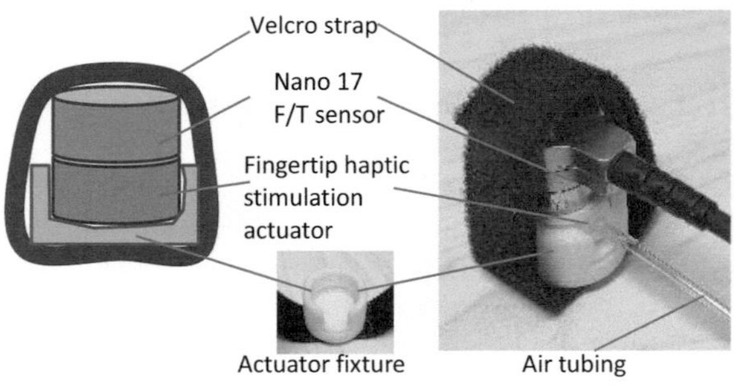

manufacturing, which was mounted on a guide rail (see Fig. 6.4b). The system response time was evaluated by generating a stimulation force that ramps up from 0 to 4 N and then returns to 0 N, with repeated tests conducted three times (Fig. 6.5).

User Experience Study

To investigate the impact of fingertip cutaneous haptic feedback on user attention during rehabilitation, a user study was conducted. Figure 6.6 presents the experimental set-up for conducting user study. The hypothesis was that merging haptic stimulation into exoskeleton-aided hand exercises could improve user participation in rehabilitation. Throughout the experiment, participants' attention levels were continuously tracked using the Brainlink Lite EEG system. This easy-to-wear, low-cost device contains three dry electrodes to record EEG signals and measure attention and relaxation levels via patented eSense algorithms. The data were processed using a ThinkGear AM (TGAM) module and reported attention and relaxation scores ranging from 1 to 100.

Thirteen healthy participants (seven males and six females) were included in the study, which consisted of three modes in the experiment:

- Exoskeleton-aided grasping without fingertip haptic stimulation
- Exoskeleton-aided grasping with fingertip haptic stimulation under a simulated glass weight of 150 g
- Exoskeleton-aided grasping with fingertip haptic stimulation under a simulated glass weight of 300 g

Each participant underwent four trials for each mode. The flexion/extension motion was performed five times per trial, with attention levels recorded once every second (1 Hz sampling rate). The experiment followed a pseudo-random sequence

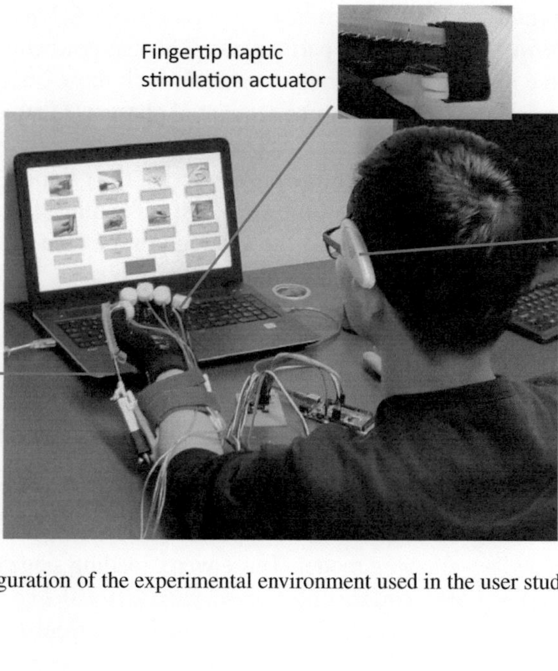

Fig. 6.6 Configuration of the experimental environment used in the user study

to minimize bias. Ethical approval for this research was obtained from the Institutional Review Board of Xi'an Jiaotong University, and written informed consent was obtained from all study participants.

Statistical Analysis

The primary outcome was the average change in attention levels across the three experimental groups. The assumptions of normality and homogeneity of variances were examined using the Shapiro–Wilk and Levene's tests, respectively. A one-way ANOVA was conducted to compare group means, with the LSD post hoc test applied to detect pairwise differences that reached statistical significance. Pairwise comparisons between experimental modes were performed using a single-tailed student t-test. The Benjamini–Hochberg procedure was employed to adjust for multiple comparisons and control the false discovery rate. A significance level of $\alpha = 0.05$ was adopted for all statistical tests. Analyses were carried out using the R programming environment (Version 3.6.3; The R Foundation).

6.6 Results

Observed Variation Pattern of Normal Contact Force

A representative normal contact force profile is displayed in Fig. 6.7, based on a single grasping trial performed by one of the participants. This pattern, which reflects the middle finger's force profile, was generally consistent with those observed in other trials. The grasping process consists of three sequential phases: (1) rapid loading, (2) gradual release, and (3) rapid release.

To characterize the normal contact force profile during the grasping process, five key parameters were defined: loading time (t_1), first unloading time (t_2), second unloading time (t_3), peak force (F_P), and the turning point of the unloading force (F_T). Summarized in Table 6.1 are the durations of these phases. While individual variations were observed in the timing of t_1, t_2 and t_3, the average phase durations across all five fingers showed consistent trends. Table 6.2 presents the peak force and unloading force data. The highest normal force observed during the grasping task was generated by the thumb. A clear descending trend in both peak and turning point forces was observed from all the five finger, indicating a gradient in force contribution across the digits.

To synchronize haptic feedback with natural grasping behavior, the actuator's stage durations were defined using the mean temporal characteristics observed across all five fingers in the glass-grasping model. These were: loading stage (t_1) = 0.36 s, first release stage (t_2) = 1.20 s, and second release stage (t_3) = 0.24 s. The fingertip haptic stimulation model was simulated under two load conditions (150 g and 300

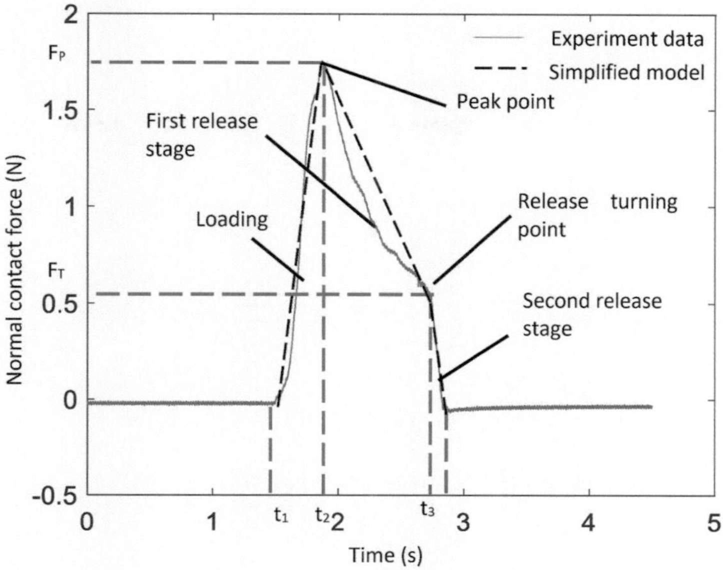

Fig. 6.7 A representative normal contact force profile during grasping. Adapted from our previous works Li et al. (2021), published under a Creative Commons CC-BY 4.0 license

Table 6.1 Duration of each stage in the glass-grasping task

Stage	Thumb (s)	Index (s)	Middle (s)	Ring (s)	Pinky (s)	Mean (s)	SD (s)
Loading time	0.35	0.3545	0.3545	0.3765	0.3725	0.3616	0.012
First release stage	1.2225	1.1705	1.195	1.223	1.146	1.1914	0.033
Second release stage	0.2155	0.253	0.2295	0.252	0.222	0.2344	0.017

g glass weights), incorporating experimentally derived mean peak forces (F_P) and unloading force turning points (F_T) to replicate realistic grasping interactions (see Table 6.3).

Results of Technical Evaluation

The haptic actuator has a weight of 2.5 ± 0.22 g and the dimensions of 16 × 16 × 20 mm. When combined with the actuator fixture, the total weight is 6.8 ± 0.23 g. The relationship between applied pressure and surface displacement, as depicted in Fig. 6.8a, reveals distinct behavioral regimes: a nonlinear response at low pressures (0–40 kPa) and a predominantly linear response at higher pressures (40–100 kPa). The curve in Fig. 6.8b, obtained by differentiating surface displacement with

Table 6.2 Peak forces and turning points during simulated glass grasping

Force	Peak force (N)–150 g	Peak force (N)–200 g	Peak force (N)–250 g	Peak force (N)–300 g	Turning point (N)–150 g	Turning point (N)–200 g	Turning point (N)–250 g	Turning point (N)–300 g
Thumb	2.1623	2.7675	3.0011	3.4288	1.3311	1.4157	1.7261	2.1491
Index	1.4373	1.3812	1.7672	1.7644	0.8035	0.8426	1.0846	1.0297
Middle	0.9966	0.9204	1.3769	1.2782	0.5544	0.4983	0.7682	0.6778
Ring	0.8528	0.929	0.8491	1.3382	0.4798	0.498	0.468	0.7503
Pinky	0.5915	0.5451	0.7081	0.7897	0.3169	0.3241	0.3848	0.4628

Table 6.3 Key force metrics in drinking glass grasping simulation

Item	Peak force (N)–150 g	Peak force (N)–300 g	Turning point force (N)–150 g	Turning point force (N)–300 g
Thumb	2.2	3.4	1.3	2.2
Index	1.4	1.8	0.8	1.0
Middle	1.0	1.3	0.6	0.7
Ring	0.9	1.3	0.5	0.8
Pinky	0.6	0.8	0.3	0.5

respect to input pressure, shows that at an input pressure close to 100 kPa, the derivative stabilizes at approximately 0.007 (indicated by the black line), with no abrupt changes. With a maximum output pressure of 100 kPa, the pneumatic proportional valve operates within the safe working limits of the actuator, as shown in the displacement–pressure characterization.

As shown in Fig. 6.8c, the distribution of force output across the actuators is nearly identical, with a roughly linear relationship between the generated force on

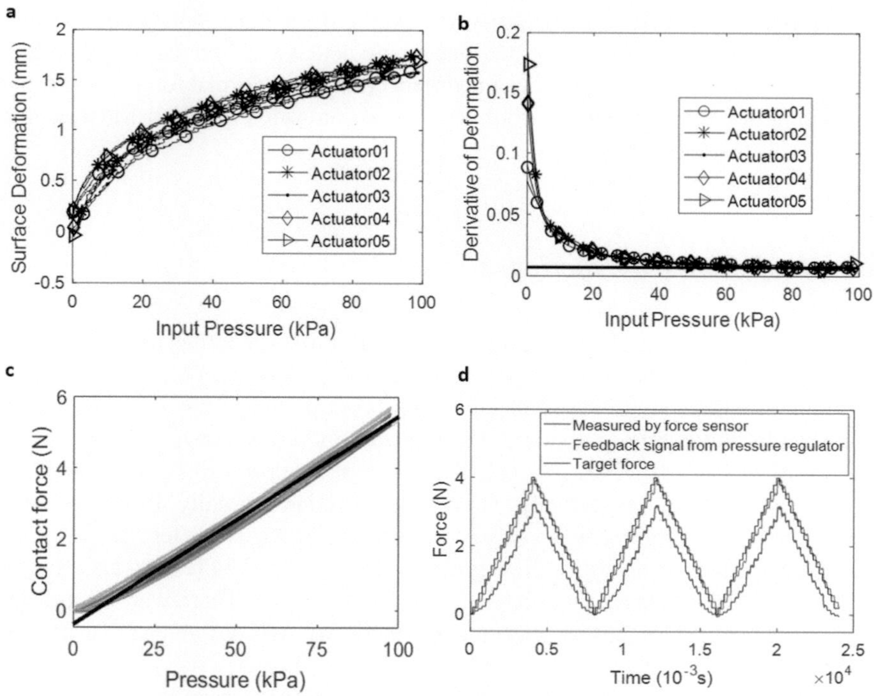

Fig. 6.8 Key experimental characterization results of the actuator system: **a** surface displacement vs. input pressure, **b** rate of change of displacement with respect to pressure, **c** contact force induced by input pressure, and **d** measured force versus target force comparison. Adapted from our previous works Li et al. (2021), published under a Creative Commons CC-BY 4.0 license

the actuator surface and the input pneumatic pressure. Between the input pneumatic pressure (P, in kPa) and the output contact force (F, in N), a fitted relationship is expressed by the following equation:

$$F = 0.0585P - 0.4055, \tag{6.1}$$

The actuator achieves a maximum output force of 5.436 N (SD = 0.171 N). Additionally, the actuators exhibit a minimal dead zone at low pressures, with a mean dead zone pressure of 4.233 kPa, suggesting that they should be pre-inflated to approximately 5 kPa before use. Overall, the actuators demonstrate consistent and stable performance, with negligible hysteresis.

As shown in Fig. 6.8d, the system's actual force output was compared with the desired force. The average latency of the haptic stimulation system was 0.17 s, and the achieved output force reached 79.5% of the target value. The discrepancy is primarily due to energy dissipation resulting from the elastic properties of the Velcro attachment, which is accounted for by compensating the input signal.

Compared to wearable fingertip haptic devices reviewed by Pacchierotti et al. (Pacchierotti et al. 2017), which have an average weight of 31.4 g, minimum dimensions of 12 × 12 × 30 mm, and a maximum continuous normal force range of 1.5 to 6.72 N (Sarakoglou et al. 2012; Prattichizzo et al. 2013; Girard et al. 2016; Chinello et al. 2015), the proposed 3D-printed pneumatic actuator is compact, lightweight. Despite its smaller size, it achieves a maximum continuous normal force comparable to existing devices, making it a competitive and innovative solution for wearable haptic feedback applications.

Results of the User Experience Study

For each trial, the mean attention level was derived from the recorded data. Figure 6.9 shows participants' attention levels throughout the user study. For each mode, 52 attention level data points were collected (4 trials per participant × 13 participants). Exoskeleton-only, 150 g glass, and 300 g glass conditions showed Shapiro–Wilk test results of ($W = 0.9748$, $p = 0.3323$), ($W = 0.9650$, $p = 0.1291$), and ($W = 0.9734$, $p = 0.2932$), respectively. They were all found normally distributed ($p > 0.05$). Variance homogeneity was also confirmed using Levene's test ($p = 0.154$). The average attention levels for these groups were 47.5 ± 12.34 (exoskeleton only), 56.1 ± 9.27 (150 g glass), and 63.6 ± 10.08 (300 g glass). There were significant differences between groups as determined by one-way ANOVA and LSD tests ($p < 0.05$).

As shown in Fig. 6.9, the haptic stimulation group demonstrated a statistically significant ($p = 0.000$) increase in attention levels compared to the exoskeleton-only group using paired t-test. Additionally, attention levels were significantly higher ($p = 0.000$) in the 300 g glass group compared to the 150 g glass group using paired t-test (Table 6.4).

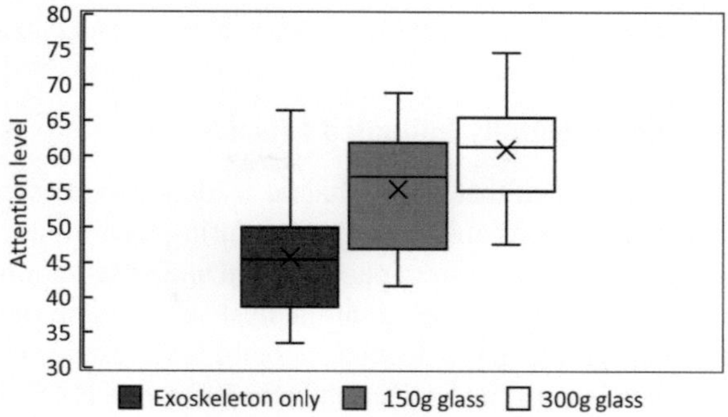

Fig. 6.9 Measured attention levels during the course of the experiment. Reformatted from our previous works (Li et al. 2021), published under a Creative Commons CC-BY 4.0 license

Table 6.4 Multiple comparison-adjusted t-test results (Benjamini–Hochberg method)

Comparison	p	Significance
E versus H (150 g)	3.820×10^{-5}	Strongly significant ($p < 0.01$)
E versus (300 g)	1.724×10^{-9}	Strongly significant ($p < 0.01$)
H 150 g versus H 300 g	5.515×10^{-6}	Strongly significant ($p < 0.01$)

E = Exoskeleton-only, H = Haptic stimulation
Reformatted from our previous works (Li et al. 2021), published under a Creative Commons CC-BY 4.0 license

6.7 Discussion and Conclusion

Discussion

The chapter described a pioneering rehabilitation system for hands, merging exoskeleton-enabled movement assistance with targeted haptic feedback on the fingertips, designed to boost patient involvement and aid in motor function restoration post-stroke. This system features fingertip haptic feedback modules composed of 3D-printed soft pneumatic actuators, in conjunction with a hand exoskeleton that combines rigid and soft elements in its mechanical structure. The haptic stimulation mimics contact forces during virtual glass-grasping motions, synchronized with the exoskeleton's assistance. The main contributions of this chapter include:

- **Integration of Fingertip Haptic Feedback**

By combining cutaneous haptic feedback at fingertips with exoskeleton-aided hand rehabilitation, the system provides simultaneous sensorimotor and tactile stimulation, enhancing engagement and recovery potential.

- **Innovative Use of Soft Material 3D Printing**

The development of low-cost, high-quality pneumatic actuators using soft material 3D printing offers rapid prototyping capabilities. Each actuator is lightweight 6.8 g

(SD = 0.23 g), compact (16 × 16 × 20 mm), and capable of generating a maximum continuous normal force of 5.4 N, comparable to existing devices.

- **Experimentally Validated Efficacy**

Tests confirmed that adding haptic feedback to exoskeleton-aided hand movements boosts user focus and participation during rehabilitation.

Regarding the system performance and observations, the actuators demonstrated stable performance with minimal hysteresis, highlighting their reliability. The addition of fingertip haptic feedback notably increased attention levels, particularly when simulating grasping heavier objects (300 g versus 150 g), suggesting that stimulation intensity positively impacts focus. These findings align with research emphasizing the role of haptic feedback in immersive training and sensory recovery (Piggott et al. 2016b).

Despite the promising results, the study identified several challenges and opportunities for improvement:

- **Miniaturization Limitations**

Current fabrication processes limit further miniaturization of the actuators. Future research should refine these processes to achieve more compact designs both for the actuators and for the pneumatic system without compromising performance.

- **Normal Force-Only Stimulation**

The system provides only normal force stimuli perpendicular to the actuator surface. While effective, the addition of tangential forces could enhance the realism of haptic feedback. However, this would increase actuator and control system complexity.

- **User Comfort and Design Optimization**

Prolonged use in rehabilitation sessions requires prioritizing user comfort and system ergonomics. Iterative design improvements, guided by patient feedback, are essential for clinical success.

- **Clinical Validation and Expanded Use Cases**

While this study focused on healthy participants, future work must include stroke patients to validate the system's clinical feasibility. The system also holds potential for broader applications, including prosthetic devices and rehabilitation for other populations, such as pediatric or geriatric patients.

- **Exploring Additional Haptic Modalities**

Future research should investigate incorporating sensations such as tangential forces, textures, or slippery interactions to provide a more vivid and realistic haptic experience.

Conclusion

This chapter presented a novel hand rehabilitation system that combines exoskeleton-assisted movements with fingertip haptic stimulation. By employing low-cost, lightweight, and high-quality 3D-printed pneumatic actuators, the system effectively enhances user engagement during training, as evidenced by increased attention levels in healthy participants. The findings suggest that adding tactile feedback to rehabilitation exercises can improve training outcomes and patient involvement.

While the study highlights the system's potential, challenges remain, including actuator miniaturization, expanding haptic modalities, and validating the system's clinical efficacy in stroke patients. Future research will address these challenges, focusing on refining actuator designs, integrating additional sensory modalities, and conducting clinical trials with diverse patient populations. This work represents a step forward in developing accessible and effective rehabilitation tools, with implications for advancing neurorehabilitation and prosthetic technology.

References

Ang BWK, Yeow C-H (2017) Print-it-Yourself (PIY) glove: A fully 3D printed soft robotic hand rehabilitative and assistive exoskeleton for stroke patients. In: 2017 IEEE/RSJ international conference on intelligent robots and systems (IROS). IEEE, pp 1219–1223

Ang KK, Guan C (2013) Brain-computer interface in stroke rehabilitation. J Comput Sci Eng 7:139–146. https://doi.org/10.5626/JCSE.2013.7.2.139

Cameirão MS, Badia SBI, Duarte E et al (2012) The combined impact of virtual reality neurorehabilitation and its interfaces on upper extremity functional recovery in patients with chronic stroke. Stroke 43:2720–2728. https://doi.org/10.1161/STROKEAHA.112.653196

Chinello F, Malvezzi M, Pacchierotti C, Prattichizzo D (2015) Design and development of a 3RRS wearable fingertip cutaneous device. In: 2015 IEEE international conference on advanced intelligent mechatronics (AIM). IEEE, pp 293–298

Girard A, Marchal M, Gosselin F et al (2016) HapTip: displaying haptic shear forces at the fingertips for multi-finger interaction in virtual environments. Front in ICT 3:00006. https://doi.org/10.3389/fict.2016.00006

Gul JZ, Sajid M, Rehman MM et al (2018) 3D printing for soft robotics–a review. Sci Technol Adv Mater 19:243–262. https://doi.org/10.1080/14686996.2018.1431862

Heo P, Gu GM, Lee SJ et al (2012) Current hand exoskeleton technologies for rehabilitation and assistive engineering. Int J Precis Eng Manufact 13:807–824. https://doi.org/10.1007/s12541-012-0107-2

Lee S, Lee K, Song C (2018) Gait training with bilateral rhythmic auditory stimulation in stroke patients: a randomized controlled trial. Brain Sci 8:164. https://doi.org/10.3390/brainsci8090164

Li M, Luo S, Nanayakkara T et al (2014a) Multi-fingered haptic palpation using pneumatic feedback actuators. Sens Actuat A Phys 218:132–141. https://doi.org/10.1016/j.sna.2014.08.003

Li M, Ranzani T, Sareh S et al (2014b) Multi-fingered haptic palpation utilizing granular jamming stiffness feedback actuators. Smart Mater Struct 23:095007. https://doi.org/10.1088/0964-1726/23/9/095007

Li M, Xu G, Xie J, Chen C (2018) A review: motor rehabilitation after stroke with control based on human intent. Proc Inst Mech Eng H 232:344–360. https://doi.org/10.1177/0954411918755828

Li M, He B, Liang Z et al (2019) An attention-controlled hand exoskeleton for the rehabilitation of finger extension and flexion using a rigid-soft combined mechanism. Front Neurorobot 13:1–13. https://doi.org/10.3389/fnbot.2019.00034

Li M, Chen J, He G et al (2021) Attention enhancement for exoskeleton-assisted hand rehabilitation using fingertip haptic stimulation. Front Robot AI 8:1–13. https://doi.org/10.3389/frobt.2021.602091

Lim S-C, Lee H-K, Park J (2014) Role of combined tactile and kinesthetic feedback in minimally invasive surgery. Int J Med Robot Comput Assist Surg 11:360–374. https://doi.org/10.1002/rcs

Minamizawa K, Prattichizzo D, Tachi S (2010) Simplified design of haptic display by extending one-point kinesthetic feedback to multipoint tactile feedback. In: 2010 IEEE haptics symposium. IEEE, pp 257–260

Momentive (2020) RTV100 Series. https://www.momentive.cn//docs/default-source/tds/snapsil/snapsil-rtv100-series-tds.pdf. Accessed 18 Jan 2025

NinjaTek (2019) Ninjaflex material properties. https://ninjatek.com/wp-content/uploads/NinjaFlex-TDS.pdf. Accessed 18 Jan 2025

Pacchierotti C, Sinclair S, Solazzi M et al (2017) Wearable haptic systems for the fingertip and the hand: taxonomy, review, and perspectives. IEEE Trans Haptics 10:580–600. https://doi.org/10.1109/TOH.2017.2689006

Piggott L, Wagner S, Ziat M (2016a) Haptic neurorehabilitation and virtual reality for upper limb paralysis: a review. Crit Rev Biomed Eng 1–2:1–32. https://doi.org/10.1615/CritRevBiomedEng.2016016046

Piggott L, Wagner S, Ziat M (2016b) Haptic neurorehabilitation and virtual reality for upper limb paralysis: a review. Crit Rev Biomed Eng 44:1–32. https://doi.org/10.1615/CritRevBiomedEng.2016016046

Prattichizzo D, Chinello F, Pacchierotti C, Malvezzi M (2013) Towards wearability in fingertip haptics: a 3-DoF wearable device for cutaneous force feedback. IEEE Trans Haptics 6:506–516. https://doi.org/10.1109/TOH.2013.53

Sagen JS, Kjeken I, Habberstad A et al (2024) Patient involvement in the rehabilitation process is associated with improvement in function and goal attainment: results from an explorative longitudinal study. J Clin Med 13:320. https://doi.org/10.3390/jcm13020320

Sarakoglou I, Garcia-Hernandez N, Tsagarakis NG, Caldwell DG (2012) A high performance tactile feedback display and its integration in teleoperation. IEEE Trans Haptics 5. https://doi.org/10.1109/TOH.2012.20

Sarkar D, D'Abbraccio J, Camboni D et al (2020) A pneumatic haptic display for collaborative robotics applications. In: 2020 IEEE international workshop on metrology for industry 4.0 & IoT. IEEE, pp 369–373

Schorr SB, Okamura AM (2017) Three-dimensional skin deformation as force substitution: wearable device design and performance during haptic exploration of virtual environments. IEEE Trans Haptics 10:418–430. https://doi.org/10.1109/TOH.2017.2672969

Secoli R, Milot M-H, Rosati G, Reinkensmeyer DJ (2011) Effect of visual distraction and auditory feedback on patient effort during robot-assisted movement training after stroke. J Neuroeng Rehabil 8:21. https://doi.org/10.1186/1743-0003-8-21

Sharififar S, Shuster JJ, Bishop MD (2018) Adding electrical stimulation during standard rehabilitation after stroke to improve motor function: a systematic review and meta-analysis. Ann Phys Rehabil Med 61:339–344. https://doi.org/10.1016/j.rehab.2018.06.005

Sigrist R, Rauter G, Riener R, Wolf P (2013) Augmented visual, auditory, haptic, and multimodal feedback in motor learning: a review. Psychon Bull Rev 20:21–53. https://doi.org/10.3758/s13423-012-0333-8

Song G, Ryu HJ (2016) Effects of gait training with rhythmic auditory stimulation on gait ability in stroke patients. J Phys Ther Sci 28:1403–1406. https://doi.org/10.1589/jpts.28.1403

Takeuchi N, Izumi S-I (2013) Rehabilitation with poststroke motor recovery: a review with a focus on neural plasticity. Stroke Res Treat 2013:128641. https://doi.org/10.1155/2013/128641

Teo WP, Chew E (2014) Is motor-imagery brain-computer interface feasible in stroke rehabilitation? PM and R 6:723–728. https://doi.org/10.1016/j.pmrj.2014.01.006

Ueki S, Kawasaki H, Ito S et al (2012) Development of a hand-assist robot with multi-degrees-of-freedom for rehabilitation therapy. IEEE/ASME Trans Mechatron 17:136–146. https://doi.org/10.1109/TMECH.2010.2090353

Yap HK, Ng HY, Yeow C-H (2016) High-force soft printable pneumatics for soft robotic applications. Soft Robot 3:144–158. https://doi.org/10.1089/soro.2016.0030

Yue Z, Zhang X, Wang J (2017) Hand rehabilitation robotics on poststroke motor recovery. Behav Neurol 2017:1–20. https://doi.org/10.1155/2017/3908135

Zhai Y, Wang Z, Kwon K et al (2021) Printing multi-material organic haptic actuators. Adv Mater 33:2002541. https://doi.org/10.1002/adma.202002541

Chapter 7
Neural and Behavioral Effects of Integrated Exoskeleton and Cutaneous Haptic Feedback in Simulated Hand Rehabilitation

Enhancing current hand rehabilitation training through additional sensory stimulation methods may contribute to improved therapeutic outcomes in stroke survivors. This chapter describes a comparative study investigating the impact of integrating exoskeleton-based hand rehabilitation with haptic stimulation on fingertips on behavioral responses and event-related brain potentials. The study also investigates the touch-induced stimulation effects induced by holding a water bottle compared to those elicited through pneumatically driven cutaneous stimulation at the fingertip. Cutaneous stimulation was synchronized with the finger motion assisted by an exoskeleton. Three configurations were compared in the experiment: (1) exoskeleton-supported grasping in the absence of haptic feedback, (2) with fingertip haptic stimulation, and (3) with a water bottle. Behavioral analysis showed no significant difference in recognition accuracy across configurations ($p = 0.658$). The presence of haptic feedback—either through dedicated actuators or a water bottle—resulted in significantly faster response times than its absence ($p = 0.006$), with no significant difference between the two feedback types ($p = 0.441$). However, with haptic stimulation, the response time was comparable to that with the water bottle with a p value of 0.441, yet notably shorter than when there was no haptic stimulation with a p value of 0.006). Event-related potential analysis indicated increased activation within the somatosensory, premotor, and primary motor regions when concurrent hand motion support and tactile feedback were delivered, with a P300 amplitude of 9.46 μV. This combination significantly improved P300 amplitude ($p = 0.006$) compared with the baseline condition of hand motion assistance without additional stimulation. No statistically significant differences were observed among the remaining mode comparisons ($p = 0.227$, $p = 0.918$). P300 latency was not strongly influenced by mode ($p = 0.102$), and also stimulation intensity did not influence P300 amplitude or latency. In conclusion, the synergistic application of exoskeleton-assisted movement and haptic feedback enhances cortical responses in motor and sensory areas of the brain. Sensory effects associated with grasping a water bottle and pneumatic fingertip actuators are comparable, offering insights for enhanced rehabilitation strategies.

M. Li and B. He, *Intention-Controlled Hand Rehabilitation for Stroke Survivors*,
https://doi.org/10.1007/978-981-95-4196-6_7

7.1 Introduction

Chapter 6 introduced the integration of cutaneous haptic stimulation at fingertips into exoskeleton-aided hand rehabilitation, demonstrating its potential to enhance engagement and support motor function restoration. Using 3D-printed pneumatic actuators, our system delivered tactile feedback during continuous passive motion (CPM) tasks, significantly improving participants' attention levels (Li et al. 2021). Building on this foundation, this chapter explores the neural and behavioral effects of integrating exoskeleton-aided hand movements with cutaneous stimulation at fingertips, focusing on both neural and behavioral outcomes.

CPM training, widely used in exoskeleton-assisted rehabilitation, involves repetitive grasping tasks to improve hand motor function. However, the inherently passive nature of CPM limits patient engagement, which is critical for restoring motor control and sensory feedback loops (Almusawi and Husi 2021). Stroke survivors often face additional challenges, such as somatosensory deficits that impair haptic and proprioceptive sensations, further hindering their rehabilitation progress (Ethier et al. 2015; Li et al. 2018; Teo and Chew 2014). These challenges underscore the importance of developing innovative approaches to enhance sensory engagement and active participation in rehabilitation.

Multimodal sensory feedback—combining visual, auditory, and haptic stimuli—has been shown to enhance motor learning, enrich sensorimotor feedback, and promote functional recovery (Norwood et al. 2023; Sharififar et al. 2018; Winkler et al. 2022). Cutaneous haptic stimulation, which directly targets mechanoreceptors in the skin, plays a vital role in improving tactile perception and engagement during rehabilitation. While Chap. 6 focused on the behavioral benefits of this approach, this chapter extends the research by investigating the neural mechanisms involved and comparing the effects of real versus virtual tactile interactions.

Event-related potentials (ERPs) derived from electroencephalographic (EEG) signals provide a powerful tool for examining brain responses to sensory stimuli. Among ERP components, the P300 is particularly relevant, as it reflects attention allocation and cognitive processing. Its amplitude and latency serve as quantitative markers for assessing neural activity (Olichney et al. 2022; Salehinejad et al. 2021). Previous studies have successfully used P300 to evaluate somatosensory responses to cutaneous haptic feedback (Chen and Ge 2017; Tang et al. 2020; Zhang et al. 2016), making it an ideal metric for this study.

This chapter presents a detailed comparison of exoskeleton-assisted hand rehabilitation combined with fingertip haptic stimulation, evaluated through both behavioral and ERP analyses. Specifically, it examines the differences between real object touch (e.g., grasping a water bottle) and fingertip haptic feedback generated by pneumatic actuators during rehabilitation tasks. Behavioral analysis focuses on stimulation recognition accuracy and response time, while ERP analysis evaluates P300 amplitude and latency. By integrating these two perspectives, the study aims to uncover the effect of synchronized motor assistance and cutaneous fingertip stimulation on brain activation patterns. This study was initially published in our previous article (Li et al. 2023), with the methods and results reorganized here for clarity and alignment with the framework introduced in Chap. 6.

Below is an outline of the remaining content in this chapter: Sect. 7.2 describes the system design, Sect. 7.3 outlines the experimental protocol, Sect. 7.4 presents the experimental results, and Sect. 7.5 provides a discussion of the findings.

7.2 Design of Hand Rehabilitation System

The combined hand rehabilitation utilizing exoskeleton-based assistance with fingertip haptic stimulation serves to enhance patient engagement during training (see Fig. 7.1a). The system is intended to (1) help rebuild the body's sensorimotor feedback system, (2) boost motor learning, and (3) support the recovery of hand movement ability. The pneumatic hand exoskeleton helps users perform grasping motions, offering both motor-sensory feedback. Simultaneously, fingertip-mounted haptic actuators produce interaction forces at the actuator-fingertip interface, thereby enhancing somatosensory input for the user. The actuators generate fingertip force that scales with the progression of the grasping motion.

The pneumatically actuated hand exoskeleton, depicted in Fig. 7.1b, consists of five air bellows (outer diameters: 15 mm and 9 mm) mounted on the backs of the fingers. These bellows are fabricated from thermoplastic polyurethane (TPU) using injection molding. All five fingers of the hand exoskeleton are actuated simultaneously through a single pneumatic channel to assist in performing a grasping motion. Weighing 120 g in total, the exoskeleton is lightweight and portable. The correlation between the pneumatic pressure (P_1) applied to the hand exoskeleton actuators and the mean metacarpophalangeal (MCP) joint bending angle (A) across all five fingers during grasping is described by the following linear equation:

$$A = \frac{3}{5} P_1, \tag{7.1}$$

where P_1 represents the air pressure within the exoskeleton's chamber in kilopascals (kPa) and A denotes the average MCP joint flexion angle in degrees. When the maximum pressure of 100 kPa is applied, the system achieves an average MCP joint angle of 60°, indicating a strong and predictable pressure-angle response.

The haptic stimulation modules are affixed to the fingertips, as depicted in Fig. 7.1c. Each actuator is equipped with an air chamber that inflates when pressurized air is introduced, generating force on the fingertip of the user. The design and fabrication procedures for these actuators were thoroughly described in our earlier study presented in Chap. 6 and (Li et al. 2021). The actuators used here are smaller than those in our prior work (height: 11 vs. 16 mm, length: 16 vs. 20 mm). These actuators are capable of generating a contact force of up to 12 N. The correlation between the pneumatic pressure (P_2) and the resulting output force (F) is given by:

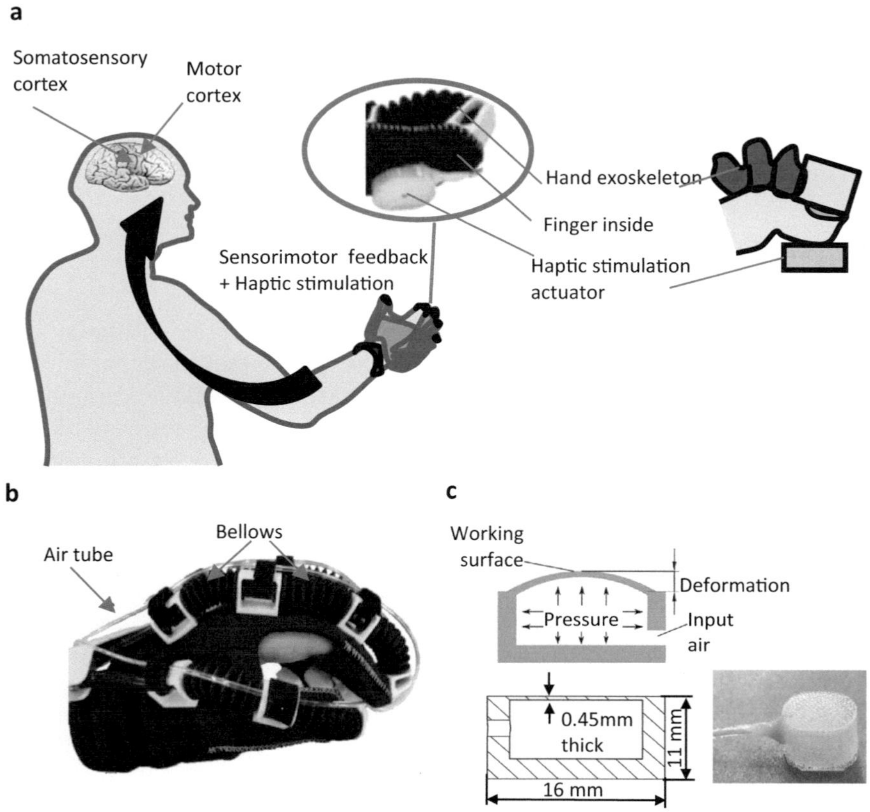

Fig. 7.1 Diagrams depicting: **a** the integrated hand rehabilitation robot comprising a hand exoskeleton and fingertip haptic feedback module, **b** the mechanical structure of the hand exoskeleton, and **c** the design of the pneumatic actuator for fingertip haptic stimulation. Reformatted from our previous work (Li et al. 2023), published under a Creative Commons CC BY 4.0 license

$$F = 0.03767P_2 - 0.1694, \tag{7.2}$$

where P_2 (in kPa) represents the pressure inside the haptic actuator's air chamber, and F (in N) denotes the force applied to the fingertip.

Figure 7.2 illustrates the system integration and control architecture of the proposed device. Compressed air was supplied by a U-STAR601 air pump (U-STAR, China). Upon receiving a start command from the computer, the JY-DAM10AIAO analog I/O module (Beijing Elit Gathering Electron, Beijing, China) sends control signals to the pressure adjustment modules, which manage the air pressure in the hand exoskeleton. The desired haptic force at the fingertip is calculated based on a linear correlation between fingertip force and grasping motion. This calculated force is transferred to the analog I/O module, which adjusts the pneumatic pressure within the haptic feedback actuators through the use of pressure adjustment modules

(SMC ITV0010). Feedback from the pressure adjustment modules is monitored by the analog I/O module.

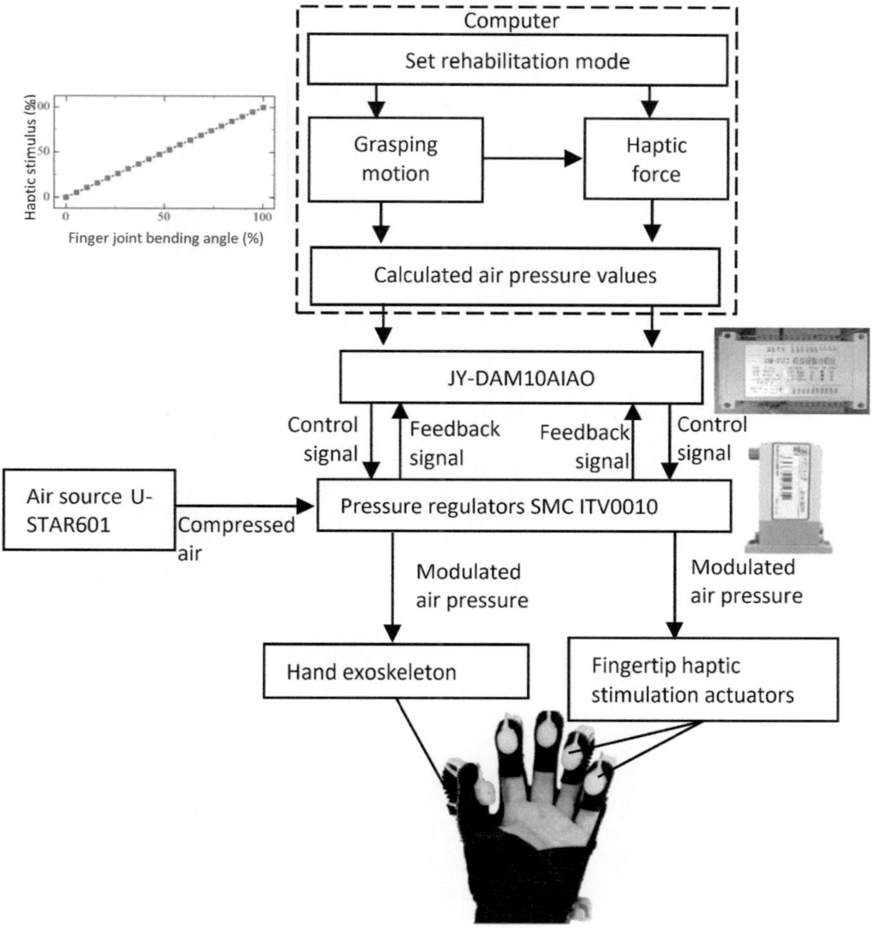

Fig. 7.2 System integration and control. Reformatted from our previous work (Li et al. 2023), published under a Creative Commons CC BY 4.0 license

7.3 Experimental Protocol

Experimental Design

This research seeks to investigate how the integration of fingertip haptic feedback and motor signaling influences the underlying neural substrates, and to evaluate how differing intensities of haptic stimulation modulate cortical activity. To achieve this, we designed a controlled experiment focusing solely on skin-based haptic stimulation at the fingertips as the independent variable, and analyzed behavioral data and event-related potentials (ERPs) from participants across three experimental conditions. The experimental conditions are as follows: (1) grasping movement facilitated by the exoskeleton with no fingertip haptic stimulation, (2) grasping movement facilitated by the exoskeleton with fingertip haptic stimulation, and (3) grasping movement facilitated by the exoskeleton performed with a water bottle. In condition (2), haptic stimulation at the fingertip is triggered as soon as the exoskeleton is activated. In condition (3), the haptic stimulation starts when the fingertips make contact with the water bottle.

In rehabilitation mediated by virtual reality (VR), patients typically perform tasks that involve grasping virtual objects. When interacting with these objects, corresponding haptic feedback is generated to simulate the sensation of touching real-world objects. The act of grasping a water bottle represents a fundamental daily task and is frequently incorporated into VR rehabilitation protocols. Hence, condition (3) was designed to compare the cutaneous sensations generated by grasping a real water bottle with those generated by fingertip cutaneous haptic feedback.

Experimental Platform

Figure 7.3a illustrates the setup configuration of the test system. Throughout the test, EEG signals of the participants were continuously recorded at a sampling rate of 1 kHz utilizing a 64-channel EEG system (Neuroscan Quik-Cap, Compumedics Limited, Victoria, Australia). The experimental platform was controlled by custom software developed in E-Prime (Psychology Software Tools, Sharpsburg, USA) and CURRY 7 (Compumedics Limited, Victoria, Australia), as depicted in Fig. 7.3b.

Since ERPs occur several hundred milliseconds after stimulation, accurate timing of stimulus events is crucial. To achieve this, when activation of the pneumatic haptic actuator or exoskeleton is required, the software transmits a control signal to the DAM module, marking the start of stimulation. Similarly, when the stimulation ends, a command is sent to mark its conclusion. Behavioral data, including keystroke responses and reaction times, are recorded during the experiment.

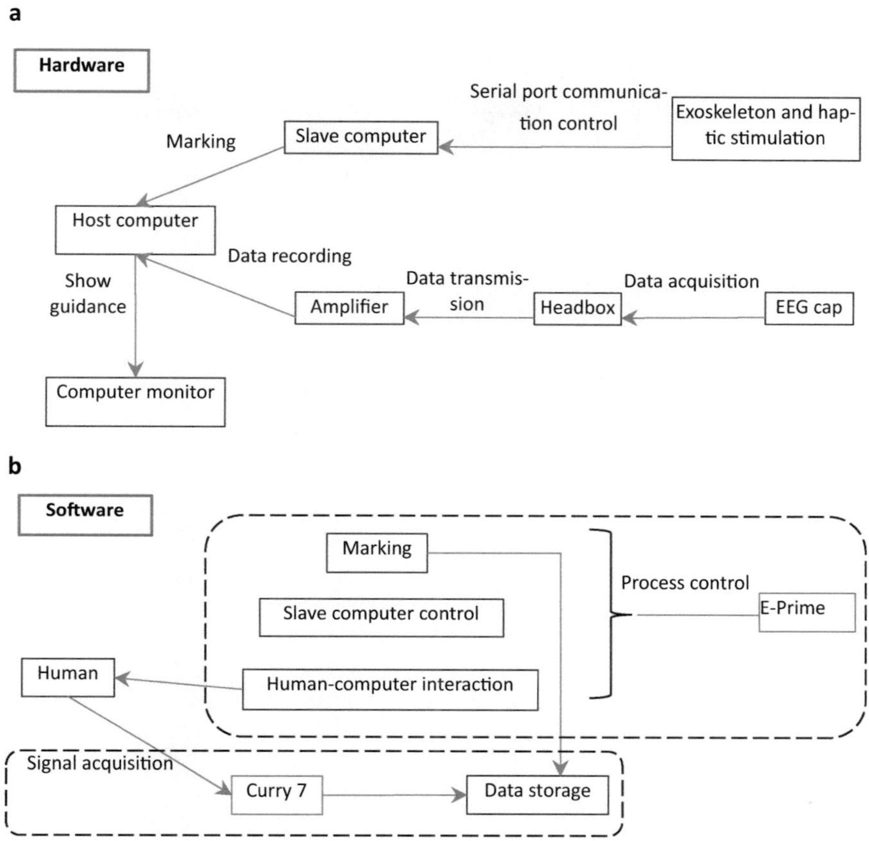

Fig. 7.3 The test system: **a** hardware architecture and **b** software architecture

Experimental Setup and Procedure

The experimental setup is shown in Fig. 7.4a and the experimental procedure is outlined in Fig. 7.4b. Three levels of fingertip cutaneous stimulation were used, as detailed in Table 7.1. As shown in the table, the mean contact forces at the fingertips in condition (3) (water bottle grasping) were slightly higher than those in condition (2) (haptic stimulation), though the difference was minimal. For this reason, we consider the contact forces in conditions (2) and (3) to be comparable across the different stimulation levels. In our previous study presented in Chap. 6 and (Li et al. 2021), we measured the contact forces at the fingertips during the grasping of a glass, finding that the average peak forces ranged from 0.59 to 3.43 N when grasping glasses of varying weights (150 to 300 g). The fingertip contact forces in this study fall within that range.

Eight healthy participants took part in this study, all of whom were right-handed males (average age: 24.5) with no prior experience using the proposed system. Prior

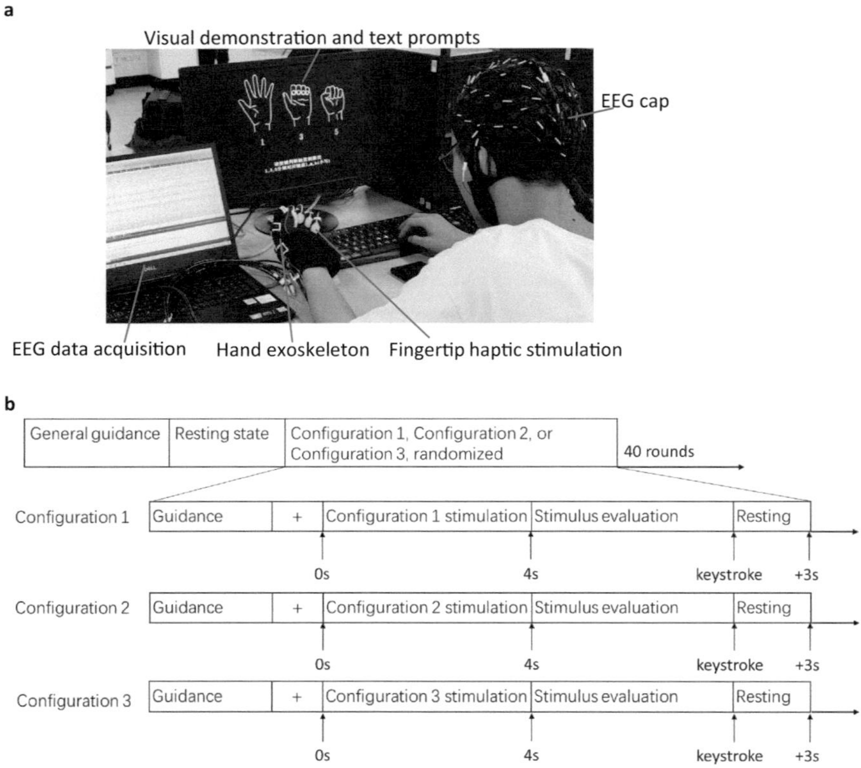

Fig. 7.4 **a** Experimental set-up and **b** experimental procedure. Reformatted from our previous work (Li et al. 2023), published under a Creative Commons CC BY 4.0 license

Table 7.1 Stimulation intensity levels used in the experiment

Levels of stimulation intensity	Low	Medium	High
Hand exoskeleton air pressure (kPa)	20	60	100
Average MCP joint bending angle (°)	12	36	60
Haptic actuator air pressure (kPa)	20	60	100
Mean fingertip contact force (Configuration 2) (N)	0.84	2.4	3.67
Mean fingertip contact force (Configuration 3) (N)	1.48	2.61	3.84

Reformatted from our previous work (Li et al. 2023), published under a Creative Commons CC BY 4.0 license

to the experiment, participants familiarized themselves with the stimulation levels. This familiarization involved presenting the three experimental configurations and their respective stimulation levels, and repeating the process five times. As shown in Fig. 7.4a, each participant wore the exoskeleton on their left hand in the experiment. The experiment began after recording participant information and providing general instructions on a computer monitor. Participants then pressed a key to begin collecting baseline EEG data while they were instructed to remain relaxed and as still as possible. Once the baseline data were collected, participants pressed a key to proceed to the main experimental phase.

A visual prompt appeared on the computer monitor before each stimulus was presented. Participants were instructed to remain still and refrain from blinking until the prompt disappeared, after which they selected the intensity level by pressing the respective keys ('l', 'm', or 'h' for low, medium, and high, respectively). The maximum duration of each stimulus was four seconds. When the participant responded by pressing a key, or the preset time limit was achieved, the haptic stimulation was then deactivated, and also the pneumatic exoskeleton was returned to its initial state. A three-second resting period followed before the next stimulus. Each trial involved the presentation of all three stimulation levels, randomly ordered. The experiment was conducted 40 times, with a longer break (up to 30 min) provided after every five rounds.

7.4 Methods for Analyzing Experimental Data

A dual analytical approach was employed, encompassing behavioral assessment and ERP analysis to examine the effects of combining hand rehabilitation facilitated by an exoskeleton with fingertip haptic stimulation. The behavioral analysis focused on two key measures: reaction duration and identification precision. Identification precision was determined by the proportion of accurately recognized stimulation levels relative to the overall number of stimulations. Reaction duration was characterized as the temporal gap between the display of the selection interface on the screen and the participant's keypress. Trials in which participants misidentified the stimulation level were excluded from the analysis.

The ERP analysis focused on assessing the latency and amplitude of the P300 component. The EEG data were preprocessed to eliminate artifacts and noise. Specifically, EEG signals were recorded using 64 channels, although channels CB1 and CB2 (non-standard Neuroscan channels not part of the 10–20 system), along with reference channels M1 and M2, were excluded from further analysis. A bandpass filter of 1–40 Hz was applied to reduce power-line interference and other noise. Based on stimulation markers, the EEG data were segmented into 130 epochs in total. Of these, 10 epochs represented the resting state, while the remaining 120 corresponded to trials involving low, medium, and high stimulation levels. A baseline correction was then applied to the 120 stimulation-related epochs using data collected 1000 ms before stimulus onset. Independent Component Analysis (ICA) was applied to remove artifacts caused by eye movements, head movements, and muscle activity.

In this study, R software (Version 4.2.2) was used for all statistical analyses, with a significance level set at $p < 0.05$. To evaluate the normality of the data, the Shapiro–Wilk test was first performed. If the data were found to be non-normally distributed, a Friedman test was used to examine differences across groups. The assumption of homogeneity of variance for normally distributed data was tested through Levene's test, followed by ANOVA to determine group differences. Two-tailed t-tests were employed for pairwise comparisons. In cases involving multiple tests, the false discovery rate was controlled using the Benjamini–Hochberg correction.

7.5 Results

Recognition Accuracy of the Stimulation

Figure 7.5 presents the recognition accuracy across varied stimulation intensities. The highest accuracy was observed for low-level stimulation, whereas the lowest accuracy occurred with medium-level stimulation, accompanied by notable individual variability. Due to the lack of normality confirmation across all datasets, a Friedman test was conducted. The results showed no significant differences in recognition accuracy between experimental configurations ($p = 0.658$), suggesting that the type of experimental mode did not have a significant impact on performance. However, statistically significant differences were found in recognition accuracy across stimulation levels within Configuration 1 ($p = 0.015$), particularly between the medium and low levels ($p = 0.005$). Similarly, Configuration 2 also revealed significant differences ($p = 0.028$), while no such differences were detected in Configuration 3 ($p = 0.093$). Configuration 2's medium and low stimulation levels had significant differences in accuracy with a p value of 0.025.

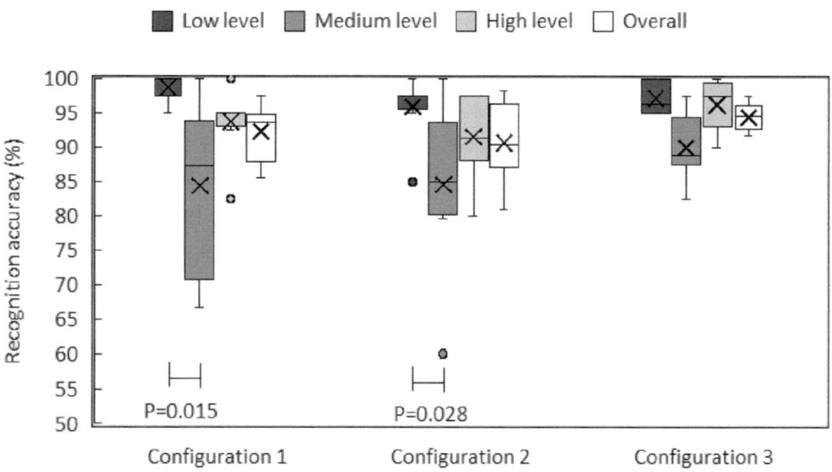

Fig. 7.5 Recognition accuracies across stimulation levels. Reformatted from our previous work (Li et al. 2023), published under a Creative Commons CC BY 4.0 license

Response Time

Figure 7.6 illustrates the mean response time for participants in identifying the stimulation level. Participants responded most quickly to the low stimulation level across all three experimental configurations (472.9, 399.2, and 413.4 ms for Configuration 1, 2 and 3, respectively), whereas they took the longest to respond to the high stimulation level (609.0, 519.8, and 467.3 ms for Configuration 1, 2 and 3, respectively). The overall mean response time was shortest in Configuration 3 (433.1 ms) and longest in Configuration 1 (521.8 ms). Given that normality was established for all samples and homogeneity of variance was confirmed (Levene test $p = 0.308$), a multi-factor ANOVA was performed. The results indicated that both stimulation intensities ($p = 0.005$) and experimental configurations ($p = 0.001$) significantly influenced response time, with no significant interaction between these two factors ($p = 0.948$). Significant differences were noted between the high and low stimulation levels, as well as between high and medium levels, but not between medium and low levels (p values were 0.000, 0.001, and 0.070, respectively). Pairwise comparisons revealed substantial differences between Configuration 1 and Configuration 2, and Configuration 1 and Configuration 3, while no difference was observed between Configuration 2 and Configuration 3 (p values were 0.018, 0.000, and 0.441, respectively). In conclusion, the response time was notably reduced when exoskeleton-assisted grasping was combined with haptic stimulation at fingertips, compared to scenarios where only exoskeleton-aided grasping was utilized.

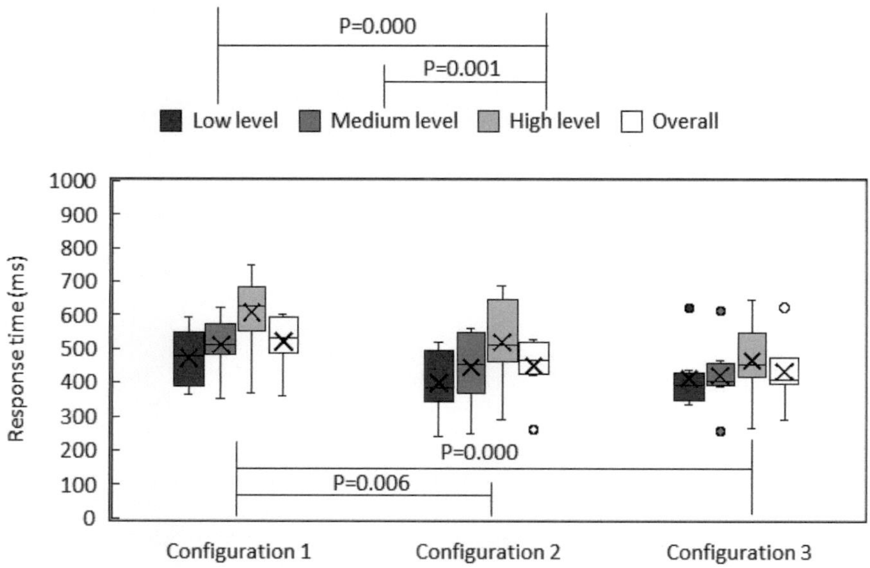

Fig. 7.6 Response time for stimulation level recognition. Reformatted from our previous work (Li et al. 2023), published under a Creative Commons CC BY 4.0 license

ERP Analysis

ERP data demonstrated distinct P300 components throughout the brain for all participants under all conditions. The mean P300 amplitude at the FCZ channel across the three configurations is depicted in Fig. 7.7a. As illustrated in subfigure a of Fig. 7.8, 7.9, and 7.10, Configuration 2 exhibited the highest P300 amplitude (9.46 μV), followed by Configuration 1 (7.41 μV) and Configuration 3 (6.98 μV). The shortest P300 latency was observed in Configuration 2 (433 ms), with Configuration 3 showing a slightly longer latency (449 ms), and Configuration 1 having the longest latency (459 ms). The topographical P300 maps (refer to subfigure b in Figs. 7.7, 7.8, 7.9, and 7.10) highlight the most extensive and robust activation in the CPZ-FZ region, particularly prominent in Configuration 2 (see Fig. 7.9a). This suggests enhanced activation of the primary somatosensory cortex (S1), premotor cortex (PM), and primary motor cortex (M1), when both exoskeleton-based hand motion assistance and fingertip haptic stimulation were provided.

Figure 7.11 presents P300 amplitude and latency across experimental conditions. Our statistical analyses indicated that the P300 amplitude data followed a normal distribution (with *p*-values of 0.223, 0.521, and 0.133), whereas the P300 latency data

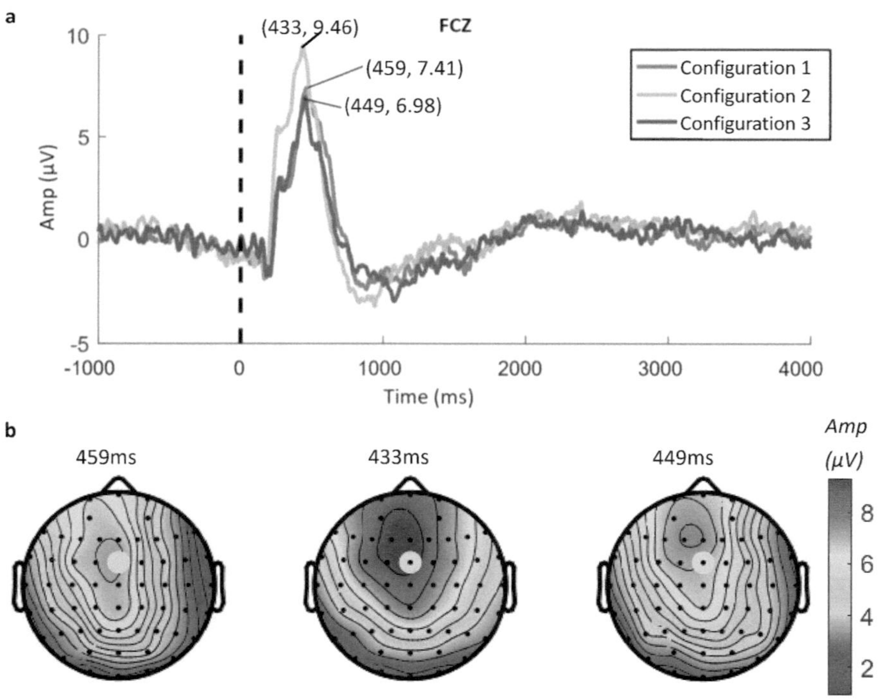

Fig. 7.7 Average data of the three configurations: **a** grand average P300 waveform recorded at the FCz electrode and **b** scalp topography of P300 amplitude at its peak latency. Reformatted from our previous work (Li et al. 2023), published under a Creative Commons CC BY 4.0 license

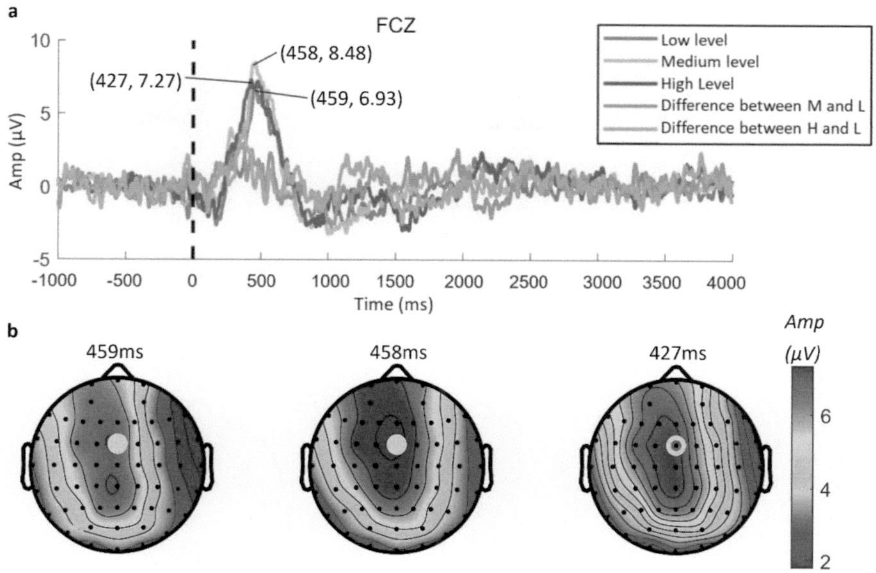

Fig. 7.8 Data of configuration 1: **a** grand average P300 waveform recorded at the FCz electrode and **b** scalp topography of P300 amplitude at its peak latency. Reformatted from our previous work (Li et al. 2023), published under a Creative Commons CC BY 4.0 license

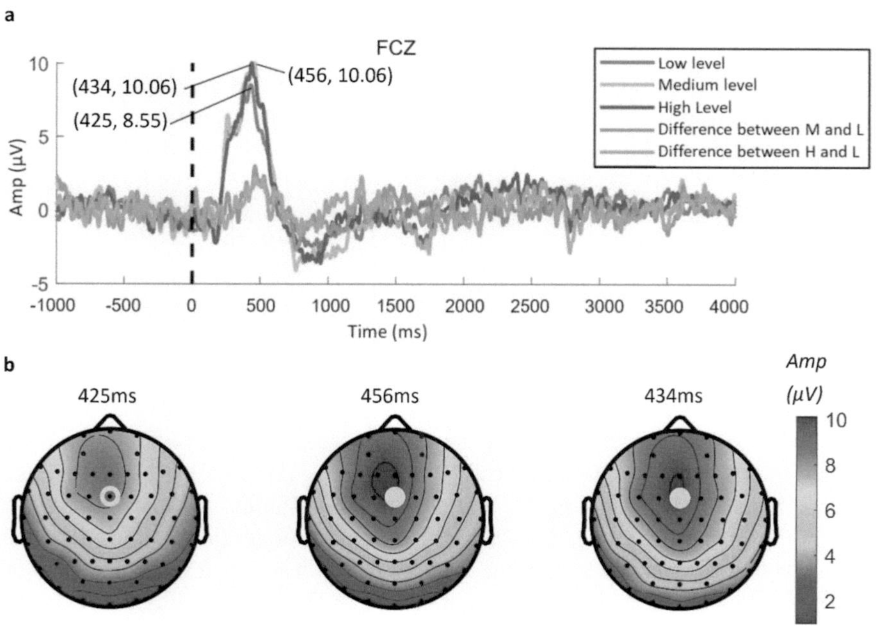

Fig. 7.9 Data of configuration 2: **a** grand average P300 waveform recorded at the FCz electrode and **b** scalp topography of P300 amplitude at its peak latency. Reformatted from our previous work (Li et al. 2023), published under a Creative Commons CC BY 4.0 license

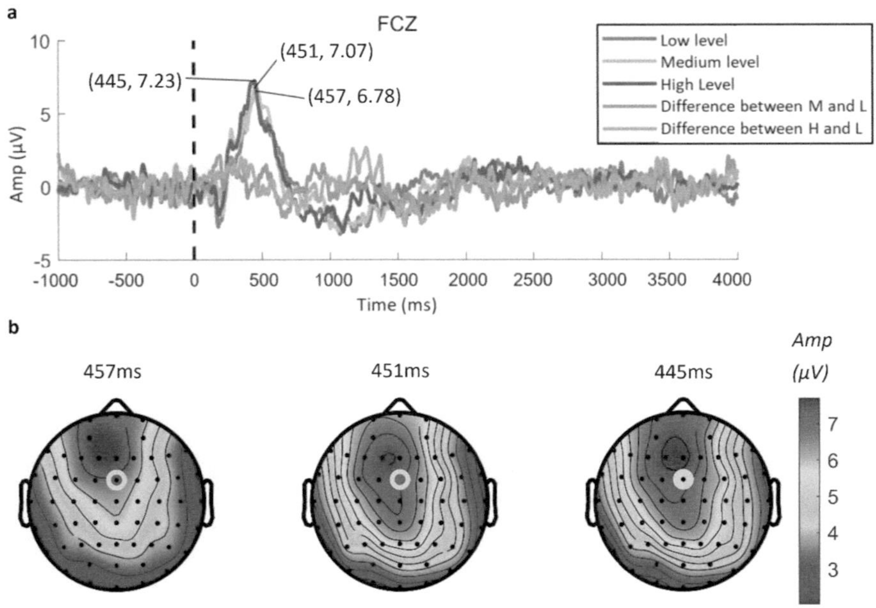

Fig. 7.10 Data of configuration 3: **a** grand average P300 waveform recorded at the FCz electrode and **b** scalp topography of P300 amplitude at its peak latency. Reformatted from our previous work (Li et al. 2023), published under a Creative Commons CC BY 4.0 license

did not (with *p*-values of 0.007, 0.161, and 0.011). The assumption of homogeneity of variance for P300 amplitudes was met with the *p* value of 0.965. P300 amplitude was significantly enhanced in Configuration 2 relative to Configuration 1, as indicated by a Student's t-test ($p = 0.006$). However, no significant differences were observed between Configurations 2 and 3 ($p = 0.227$) or between Configurations 1 and 3 ($p = 0.918$). This suggests that integrating exoskeleton-assisted hand motion with fingertip haptic feedback elicited a stronger P300 response than using exoskeleton motion alone. In contrast, the response to haptic feedback and the water bottle appeared similar. The Friedman test indicated that the experimental configurations did not significantly influence P300 latency ($p = 0.102$).

Further in-group analyses showed that different stimulation levels within the same mode had no significant effect on P300 amplitude or latency. For Configuration 1, the medium intensity produced the highest P300 amplitude (8.48 μV), followed by high (7.27 μV) and low levels (6.93 μV), while latency was shortest for high stimulation (427 ms) and longest for low stimulation (459 ms). Configuration 2 showed similar results, with no significant differences between medium and high stimulation (10.06 μV), and the shortest latency for low stimulation (425 ms). In Configuration 3, the high stimulation level produced the highest amplitude (7.23 μV), and the shortest latency (445 ms). Detailed statistical results are provided in Table 7.2.

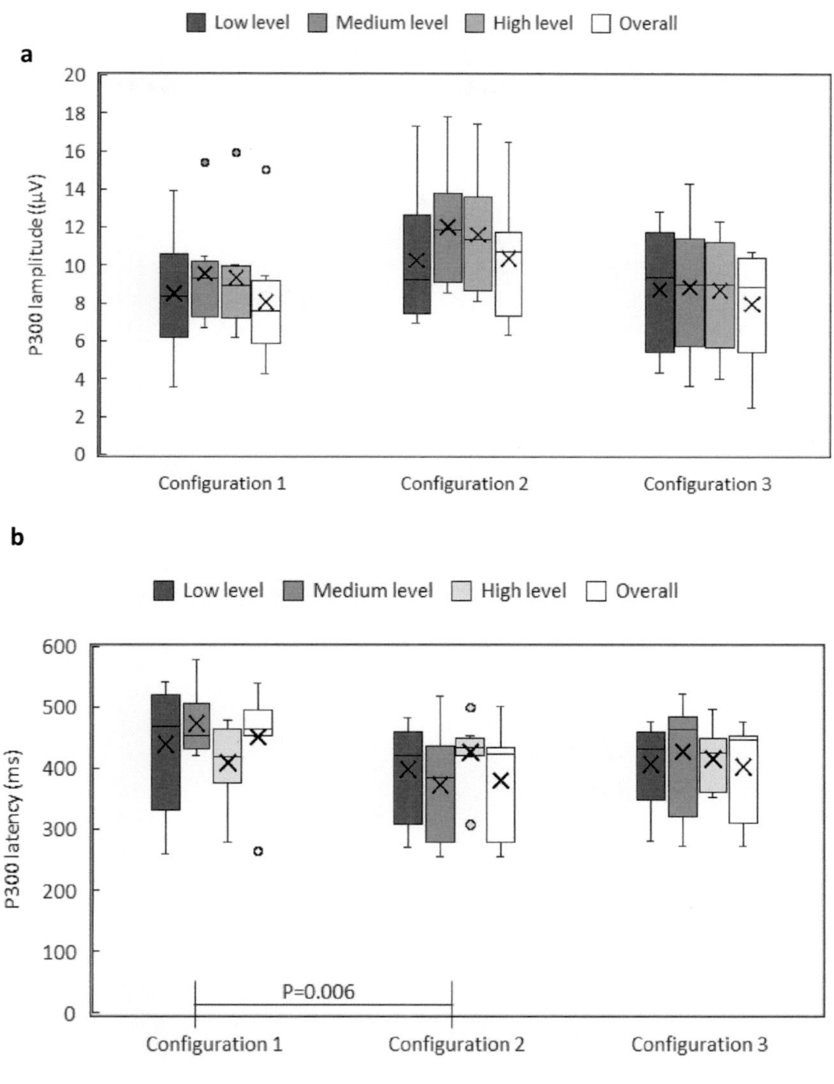

Fig. 7.11 P300 amplitude, shown in **a**, and latency, shown in **b**, at the FCz electrode across the three experimental configurations. Reformatted from our previous work (Li et al. 2023), published under a Creative Commons CC BY 4.0 license

Table 7.2 Summary of statistical comparison of P300 amplitude and latency across various stimulation levels and experimental configurations

Experimental item	Assumption of normality	Assumption of homogeneity of variance	Test used	Test result
Configuration 1 amplitude	Confirmed (p = 0.998, p = 0.067, p = 0.074)	Confirmed (p = 0.920)	One-way ANOVA (p = 0.295)	No significant difference
Configuration 1 latency	Not confirmed (p = 0.048, p = 0.153, p = 0.311)	Not applicable	Friedman test (p = 0.417)	No significant difference
Configuration 2 amplitude	Confirmed (p = 0.206, p = 0.265, p = 0.612)	Confirmed (p = 0.944)	One-way ANOVA (p = 0.414)	No significant difference
Configuration 2 latency	Not confirmed (p = 0.037, p = 0.739, p = 0.033)	Not applicable	Friedman test (p = 0.197)	No significant difference
Configuration 3 amplitude	Confirmed (p = 0.520, p = 0.959, p = 0.354)	Confirmed (p = 0.932)	One-way ANOVA (p = 0.867)	No significant difference
Configuration 3 latency	Not confirmed (p = 0.196, p = 0.018, p = 0.626)	Not applicable	Friedman test (p = 0.607)	No significant difference

7.6 Discussion and Conclusion

Discussion

The primary somatosensory cortex (S1) and motor cortex (M1) are functionally interdependent (Gómez et al. 2021). After a stroke, disruption of the motor-perception loop impairs both sensory and motor functions, which can worsen hand motor dysfunction (Edwards et al. 2019). Clinical studies indicate that cortical activity from somatosensory input can be a predictor of motor recovery (Baniqued et al. 2021). This underscores the importance of combining sensory stimulation, such as visual and tactile feedback, with motor rehabilitation during stroke recovery (He et al. 2022).

Our proposed approach, which integrates fingertip haptic feedback with exoskeleton-supported hand movement, is designed to boost neural activity in motor and sensory regions of the brain. Earlier research indicated that merging haptic feedback with exoskeleton-aided hand rehabilitation notably elevated participants' focus, possibly leading to better training results. This investigation builds upon our prior work by examining the impact of various experimental setups, including exoskeleton-assisted grasping without haptic stimulation, with haptic feedback, and with a water bottle. The findings reveal that incorporating haptic feedback alongside exoskeleton-supported hand motion considerably amplifies cortical engagement, especially in M1, PM, and S1 areas.

However, it should be noted that this study does not yet link enhanced cortical activation with improved motor function in stroke patients. Clinical studies will be necessary to further explore this connection. Our results suggest that integrating haptic stimulation with exoskeleton training may strengthen the motor-perception loop, potentially accelerating rehabilitation. The study also suggests that the touch sensations created by a water bottle and fingertip haptic feedback are comparable in their stimulation effects, which may have implications for VR-mediated rehabilitation.

In future studies, it will be crucial to investigate the long-term effects of synchronized haptic and motor feedback on stroke patients' functional recovery. The impact of different stimulation intensities on various age groups, particularly older patients with impaired tactile sensitivity.

Conclusion

This chapter investigated the combined impact of exoskeleton-based hand rehabilitation and haptic stimulation at fingertips on enhancing motor and sensory cortical activity during stroke recovery. Through a comprehensive analysis involving both behavioral metrics (recognition accuracy and response time) and ERP (event-related potentials) data, we demonstrated that integrating haptic feedback with exoskeleton-assisted hand movements has a measurable impact on brain activity and participant performance.

Our findings indicate that while the experimental configurations did not significantly alter recognition accuracy, the inclusion of haptic stimulation notably improved response time and P300 amplitude, reflecting enhanced sensory and motor cortex engagement. The ERP analysis highlighted greater activation in key brain regions such as the M1, PM, and S1 when both hand movement support and fingertip haptic feedback at the fingertips were utilized. Importantly, the P300 amplitude was significantly higher when haptic stimulation was included, suggesting that the combination of haptic feedback at fingertips and exoskeleton-aided motion creates increased stimulation intensity in both the sensory and motor areas of the brain.

Although the current study provides valuable insights into the stimulation enhancement effects, further clinical investigations are required to connect these findings with tangible improvements in hand function in stroke patients. Future research should also explore the influence of stimulation intensity, age-related factors, and additional EEG analysis techniques to better understand the mechanisms at play and refine the application of haptic exoskeleton systems in rehabilitation.

In summary, this work supports the potential of haptic-assisted exoskeletons as a powerful tool for stroke rehabilitation, offering a non-invasive method to enhance brain activation, promote motor and sensory recovery, and possibly improve rehabilitation outcomes. Further refinement and clinical validation are needed to translate these promising results into practical, effective treatments for stroke survivors.

References

Almusawi H, Husi G (2021) Design and development of Continuous Passive Motion (CPM) for fingers and wrist grounded-exoskeleton rehabilitation system. Appl Sci 11:815. https://doi.org/10.3390/app11020815

Baniqued PDE, Stanyer EC, Awais M et al (2021) Brain–computer interface robotics for hand rehabilitation after stroke: a systematic review. J Neuroeng Rehabil 18:15. https://doi.org/10.1186/s12984-021-00820-8

Chen S, Ge S (2017) Experimental research on the tactile perception from fingertip skin friction. Wear 376–377:305–314. https://doi.org/10.1016/j.wear.2016.11.014

Edwards LL, King EM, Buetefisch CM, Borich MR (2019) Putting the "sensory" into sensorimotor control: the role of sensorimotor integration in goal-directed hand movements after stroke. Front Integr Neurosci 13:00016. https://doi.org/10.3389/fnint.2019.00016

Ethier C, Gallego JA, Miller L (2015) Brain-controlled neuromuscular stimulation to drive neural plasticity and functional recovery. Curr Opin Neurobiol 33:95–102. https://doi.org/10.1016/j.conb.2015.03.007

Gómez LJ, Dooley JC, Sokoloff G, Blumberg MS (2021) Parallel and serial sensory processing in developing primary somatosensory and motor cortex. J Neurosci 41:3418–3431. https://doi.org/10.1523/JNEUROSCI.2614-20.2021

He B, Li M, He G (2022) Hand rehabilitation modes combining exoskeleton-assisted training with tactile feedback for hemiplegia patients: a preliminary study. In: Liu H, Yin Z, Liu L et al (eds) Lecture notes in computer science (including subseries Lecture Notes in Artificial Intelligence and Lecture Notes in Bioinformatics). Springer, Cham, pp 661–669

Li M, Xu G, Xie J, Chen C (2018) A review: motor rehabilitation after stroke with control based on human intent. Proc Inst Mech Eng H 232:344–360. https://doi.org/10.1177/0954411918755828

Li M, Chen J, He G et al (2021) Attention enhancement for exoskeleton-assisted hand rehabilitation using fingertip haptic stimulation. Front Robot AI 8:1–13. https://doi.org/10.3389/frobt.2021.602091

Li M, Chen J, He B et al (2023) Stimulation enhancement effect of the combination of exoskeleton-assisted hand rehabilitation and fingertip haptic stimulation. Front Neurosci 17:1149265. https://doi.org/10.3389/fnins.2023.1149265

Norwood MF, Lakhani A, Watling DP et al (2023) Efficacy of multimodal sensory therapy in adult acquired brain injury: a systematic review. Neuropsychol Rev 33:693–713. https://doi.org/10.1007/s11065-022-09560-5

Olichney J, Xia J, Church KJ, Moebius HJ (2022) Predictive power of cognitive biomarkers in neurodegenerative disease drug development: utility of the P300 event-related potential. Neural Plast 2022:1–13. https://doi.org/10.1155/2022/2104880

Salehinejad MA, Wischnewski M, Ghanavati E et al (2021) Cognitive functions and underlying parameters of human brain physiology are associated with chronotype. Nat Commun 12:4672. https://doi.org/10.1038/s41467-021-24885-0

Sharififar S, Shuster JJ, Bishop MD (2018) Adding electrical stimulation during standard rehabilitation after stroke to improve motor function: a systematic review and meta-analysis. Ann Phys Rehabil Med 61:339–344. https://doi.org/10.1016/j.rehab.2018.06.005

Tang W, Liu R, Shi Y et al (2020) From finger friction to brain activation: tactile perception of the roughness of gratings. J Adv Res 21:129–139. https://doi.org/10.1016/j.jare.2019.11.001

Teo WP, Chew E (2014) Is motor-imagery brain-computer interface feasible in stroke rehabilitation? PM and R 6:723–728. https://doi.org/10.1016/j.pmrj.2014.01.006

Winkler P, DeMarch E, Campbell H, Smith M (2022) Use of real-time multimodal sensory feedback home program improved backward stride and retention for people with Parkinson Disease: a pilot study. Clin Park Relat Disord 6:100132. https://doi.org/10.1016/j.prdoa.2022.100132

Zhang D, Xu F, Xu H et al (2016) Quantifying different tactile sensations evoked by cutaneous electrical stimulation using electroencephalography features. Int J Neural Syst 26:1–16. https://doi.org/10.1142/S0129065716500064

Chapter 8
Summary and Conclusions

Throughout the preceding chapters, we have delved into a spectrum of innovative approaches designed to enhance motor recovery and redefine rehabilitation paradigms: from soft wearable hand robots and bilateral EMG-guided systems to tau-jerk optimized exoskeleton trajectories, low-cost EEG-integrated gamified tasks, and the synergistic integration of motion assistance with fingertip haptic stimulation. These discussions have been grounded in neurophysiological principles, supported by rigorous experimental data, theoretical analyses, and practical case studies, all aimed at addressing the multifaceted challenges of hand rehabilitation—including natural kinematics preservation, muscle synergy imbalance, cognitive-motor decoupling, and the need for adaptive, multisensory engagement. As we transition into this final chapter, we will synthesize the key findings, theoretical insights, and practical implications across these domains, distilling the overarching contributions of the research presented.

8.1 Summary

This book explores the interplay between motion assistance and haptic stimulation controlled by human intent in the context of hand rehabilitation for stroke survivors, presenting an in-depth analysis of novel therapeutic approaches. The primary focus is on developing intuitive and effective systems to aid motor recovery by leveraging neurophysiological mechanisms, robotic technologies, and sensory feedback strategies. Across its chapters, the book integrates theoretical frameworks, experimental findings, and practical applications to address the multifaceted challenges of stroke rehabilitation.

The opening chapter introduces the foundational concepts of motor rehabilitation, emphasizing the importance of understanding neuroplasticity and its role in functional recovery. The synchronization of human motor intention with timely and

M. Li and B. He, *Intention-Controlled Hand Rehabilitation for Stroke Survivors*,
https://doi.org/10.1007/978-981-95-4196-6_8

appropriate feedback emerges as a crucial factor in rehabilitation efficacy. Current challenges, such as optimizing the timing of feedback, enhancing the accuracy of motor intention detection, and designing systems that accommodate cognitive variability among patients, are thoroughly discussed. The chapter also highlights the potential of brain-computer interface (BCI) technologies in stroke rehabilitation while acknowledging the need for cost-effective and user-friendly systems. This sets the stage for exploring integrated solutions that combine intent detection, robotic assistance, and feedback mechanisms.

Subsequent chapters delve into technological innovations in wearable robotics, focusing on soft exoskeletons that align with natural hand motions. These devices prioritize safety, adaptability, and user comfort, addressing limitations of traditional rigid exoskeletons. For instance, the book presents a soft robotic glove that replicates the movements of the unimpaired hand onto the impaired hand, facilitating bilateral rehabilitation. Such systems are shown to enhance the precision of motion control while reducing response delays, offering significant benefits for hemiplegic patients. Experimental results confirm the effectiveness of these devices in supporting complex hand motions and fine motor tasks, marking a substantial advancement in assistive technology.

Attention-controlled rehabilitation methods using affordable EEG sensors are another innovation highlighted in the book. These systems foster active patient participation by requiring users to maintain specific attention thresholds for device operation. Visual guidance further augments attention, leading to improved engagement and therapeutic outcomes. The simplicity and cost-efficiency of these systems make them accessible for both clinical and home-based rehabilitation, broadening their potential impact. Importantly, the use of general attention thresholds demonstrates that personalized calibration may not always be necessary, streamlining the setup process for diverse patient populations.

The book also introduces the concept of fingertip cutaneous haptic stimulation, a pioneering approach to enhance attention during rehabilitation exercises. By synchronizing haptic feedback with hand exoskeleton motions, this method creates a more immersive training experience. Experimental findings reveal that haptic stimulation significantly improves attention levels, particularly during tasks involving heavier objects. This enhancement of user engagement is attributed to the tactile sensations provided by the lightweight, pneumatically actuated haptic devices, which are designed for simplicity and effectiveness.

A comprehensive analysis of the synergistic effects of motion assistance and haptic feedback forms a cornerstone of the book. Behavioral and neurophysiological data underscore the benefits of combining these modalities, demonstrating increased activation in the motor and sensory cortical regions. The findings suggest that this integrated approach not only improves functional outcomes but also facilitates a deeper engagement with the rehabilitation process. Notably, the book compares different modes of stimulation, concluding that the combination of exoskeleton-assisted motion and fingertip haptic feedback yields the most significant benefits for stroke recovery.

Across its chapters, the book identifies several areas for future research, including the refinement of BCI systems, the exploration of additional feedback modalities, and the investigation of long-term rehabilitation outcomes. By addressing these challenges, the field can move closer to developing comprehensive and effective solutions that meet the diverse needs of stroke survivors. The emphasis on user-centered design, clinical validation, and accessibility underscores the potential of these technologies to transform rehabilitation practices.

8.2 Conclusion

This book represents a significant contribution to the field of stroke rehabilitation, offering a comprehensive exploration of motion assistance and haptic stimulation as tools to enhance recovery. By integrating human intent control, robotic assistance, and sensory feedback, it outlines a multidisciplinary approach to addressing the complex challenges faced by stroke survivors. The findings presented across the chapters highlight the transformative potential of these technologies, paving the way for more effective, personalized, and accessible rehabilitation solutions.

One of the key takeaways is the importance of synchronizing human motor intention with feedback to trigger neuroplasticity. The book identifies critical gaps in understanding the optimal timing and integration of feedback modalities, calling for further research to refine these systems. The use of BCI technologies, particularly EEG-based interfaces, emerges as a promising avenue, although challenges related to cost, usability, and variability in patient responses remain to be addressed. The development of affordable and user-friendly BCI systems tailored to the unique needs of stroke patients is a priority for future advancements.

The book underscores the advantages of soft wearable robotics, which offer safer and more adaptable alternatives to traditional rigid exoskeletons. These devices align with natural hand motions and provide precise motion control, enhancing their effectiveness in rehabilitation settings. The introduction of a bilateral robotic glove that replicates the movements of the unimpaired hand onto the impaired hand is a notable innovation, demonstrating significant potential for improving functional outcomes in hemiplegic patients. Experimental results validate the system's effectiveness, highlighting its ability to support complex tasks and reduce response delays.

Attention-controlled rehabilitation systems using low-cost EEG sensors represent another breakthrough discussed in the book. These systems actively engage patients in therapeutic exercises, leveraging attention thresholds to initiate device operation. Visual guidance enhances this engagement, making rehabilitation sessions more interactive and effective. The simplicity and cost-efficiency of these systems make them suitable for widespread adoption, offering a practical solution for both clinical and home-based settings.

The integration of fingertip cutaneous haptic stimulation with motion assistance represents a pioneering approach to enhancing user engagement. The book demonstrates that haptic feedback not only improves attention levels but also activates motor and sensory cortical regions, contributing to better therapeutic outcomes. The lightweight and cost-effective design of the haptic devices ensures their accessibility, while the synchronization with exoskeleton motions creates an immersive rehabilitation experience. These findings highlight the potential of haptic feedback to augment traditional rehabilitation methods, making them more engaging and effective.

The synergistic effects of combining motion assistance and haptic stimulation form a central theme of the book. Neurophysiological data reveal that this integrated approach significantly enhances cortical activation, reflecting a deeper engagement with the rehabilitation process. The book's comparative analysis of different stimulation modes underscores the superiority of the combined approach, which yields the most substantial benefits for stroke recovery. These insights provide a strong foundation for future research and clinical applications.

Looking ahead, the book identifies several areas for further exploration. The refinement of BCI systems to accommodate the variability in EEG signals among stroke patients, the development of advanced feedback modalities, and the investigation of long-term outcomes are critical priorities. Additionally, the book emphasizes the need for clinical validation of these systems, including trials with diverse patient populations and extended evaluation periods. By addressing these challenges, the field can realize the full potential of these innovative technologies, offering robust and user-friendly solutions for stroke survivors.

In conclusion, this book highlights the transformative potential of motion assistance and haptic stimulation in stroke rehabilitation. By integrating human intent control, robotic assistance, and sensory feedback, it presents a multidisciplinary approach that prioritizes patient engagement, accessibility, and effectiveness. The insights and innovations outlined in this work pave the way for a new era of rehabilitation practices, with the promise of improving the quality of life for stroke survivors worldwide. Further research and clinical validation will be essential to translating these promising developments into practical and impactful treatments.